HEALTH FOR THE PACIFIC 2

Healthy Living

in Papua New Guinea

compiled by Andrew Solien

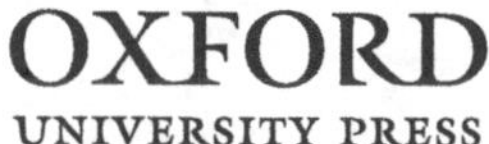

Contents

Foreword

The lack of clear, simple and accurate information about good health contributes to poor health in any society.

The Health for the Pacific series is intended to educate and highlight important health issues that are affecting the lives of Papua New Guineans.

Eating the wrong amount and kind of food contributes to ill health. Without the right amount and kind of food, two types of nutritional disorders will happen: malnutrition, namely protein-energy malnutrition, and micronutrient disorders. Therefore, there is a need to educate our people to be aware of their health, the risks to which they are exposed and the measures that must be taken to ensure adequate food intake and variety, which is essential for proper physical and mental growth for well being.

Health is everyone's concern.

I commend the compiler, Andrew Solien, Oxford University Press and the many others who have contributed to the publishing of these health books for schools in Papua New Guinea.

I trust that these books will play an important role in creating a healthy, strong and fit community for a better nation.

Dr Nicholas Mann CMS, MBBS, DCH, FACHSE

Acknowledgments

Papua New Guinea is a rich and diverse culture, with more than 700 languages spoken by its estimated 5.9 million people. It is the biggest island in the South Pacific, apart from Australia (which is also a continent) and Indonesia, with whom it shares its border.

This book is a compilation of resource materials written specifically for the education of students throughout Papua New Guinea, and for a variety of people in other institutions. Its aim is to provide education about a healthy diet, personal hygiene, the need for a clean environment at home and at school, and the importance of exercise.

I would like to thank and acknowledge the National Department of Health—in particular, Dr Greg Law—for providing technical and other resource materials. I would also like to thank the many people whom I have interviewed while compiling this book. Their time and effort has been invaluable.

Lastly, I would like to thank Oxford University Press for recognising the need to publish health materials for schools in Papua New Guinea.

Andrew Solien

Chapter 1 Why we need a healthy diet

In Papua New Guinea, food plays an important role in society. It is part of people's tradition and cultures. Food is treated with respect from the time it is planted through to the time it is eaten.

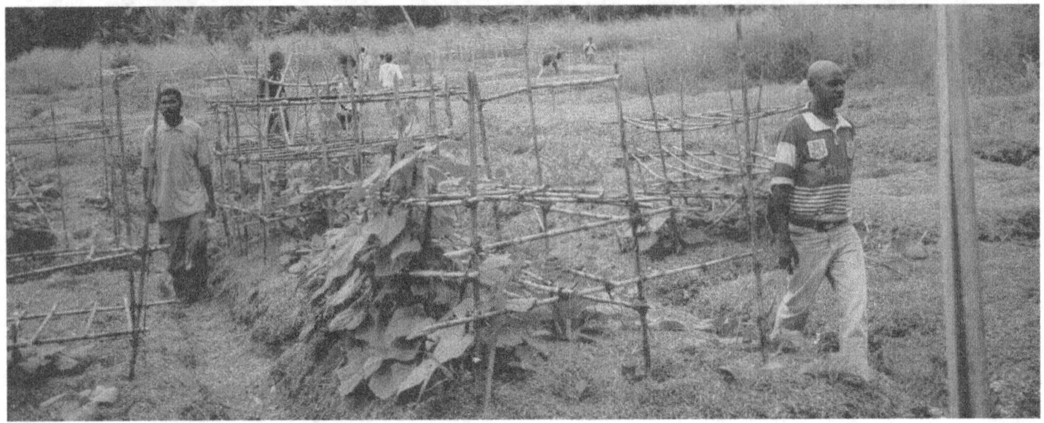

Everyone understands that food is needed so that we can live and work.

We must also understand that our health depends on the type and the amount of food we eat every day.

Healthy people eat good food. This food contains all the nutrients that our body needs to stay alive and allows us to live and work.

Everybody needs nutrients. Food contains nutrients that help our bodies to grow, give us energy, and protect us from diseases.

The Health Ministry of Papua New Guinea has a ten-year health plan, which includes a goal to improve the nutritional well being of those suffering from ill health, and to maintain the nutrition of the general population so that they will live healthier lives and contribute to the overall social and economic development of Papua New Guinea.

It also has policies for community-based nutrition services to be adopted and expanded, for maternal and child health services to support community-based monitoring of children's growth, and for nutrition centres to be established at all hospitals and district health centres.

What is nutrition?

Nutrition is the science that deals with food and how the body uses it. People, like all living things, need food to live. Food gives us the energy for every action we do, from reading a book to running a race. Food also provides substances that the body needs to build and repair its tissues and to regulate its organs and systems.

What we eat directly affects our health. A proper diet helps prevent certain illnesses and helps us to recover from others. An improper or inadequate diet increases the risk of various diseases. Eating a balanced diet is the best way to make sure that the body receives all the food substances it needs.

A balanced diet for a child

Breakfast	sweet potato dripping tinned fish green leaves	243g or 2 small 8g or 1 teaspoon 19g or 2 eating spoons 40g or small handful
Snack	ripe banana	75g or 1 small
Midday meal	sweet potato dripping tinned fish green leaves	243g or 2 small 8g or 1 teaspoon 19g or 2 eating spoons 40g or small handful
Snack	pineapple	75g or 1 slice
Evening meal	sweet potato dripping peanut flour (made from 1/4 cup peanuts) green leaves	364g or 3 small 8g or 1 teaspoon 3 eating spoons 40g or small handful

Note: a three-year-old child needs half as much protein and half as much energy as an adult. School children need as much as an adult.

A balanced diet for a Highlands person

Breakfast	sweet potato tinned dripping winged beans green leaves	425g or $3^1/_2$ small 16g or $1^1/_3$ teaspoons 40g or $^1/_6$ cup 40g or small handful
Midday meal	sweet potato tinned dripping winged beans green leaves pumpkin	425g or $3^1/_2$ small 16g or $1^1/_3$ teaspoons 40g or $^1/_6$ cup 40g or small handful 75g or $1^1/_2$ match box pieces
Evening meal	sweet potato tinned dripping winged beans green leaves pumpkin	850g or 7 small 16g or $1^1/_3$ teaspoons 40g or $^1/_6$ cup 40g or small handful 75g or $1^1/_2$ match box pieces

A balanced diet for a person living in town

Breakfast	taro margarine tinned meat green leaves	422g or 2 small 20g or $1^1/_3$ teaspoons 38g or 1 slice 40g or $^1/_3$ handful
Midday meal	taro margarine tinned meat green leaves banana	422g or 2 small 20g or $1^1/_3$ teaspoons 38g or 1 slice 40g or small handful 120g or 1 medium
Evening meal	rice margarine fresh fish green leaves banana	240g or $1^1/_4$ cups 20g or $1^1/_3$ teaspoons 100g or 1 cup 40g or small handful 180g or $1^1/_2$ medium

Your body and food

The body needs food and energy in order to work properly. Food has certain chemicals and substances called nutrients. These nutrients do one or more of these three functions:

1. they help to build, repair, or maintain body tissues
2. they help to regulate body processes
3. they provide energy.

Food is broken down through the process of digestion. Firstly, the food is chewed up in the mouth and saliva softens or moistens the starchy food for easy swallowing.

After the food is swallowed, it passes through the oesophagus, which is a tube that leads into the stomach. In the stomach, digestive juices speed up the breakdown of foods such as meat, eggs and milk.

Then the food passes from the stomach into the small intestine where the full digestion process is completed. In the small intestine, the food is completely broken down so that it can pass through the walls of the intestine and into the blood.

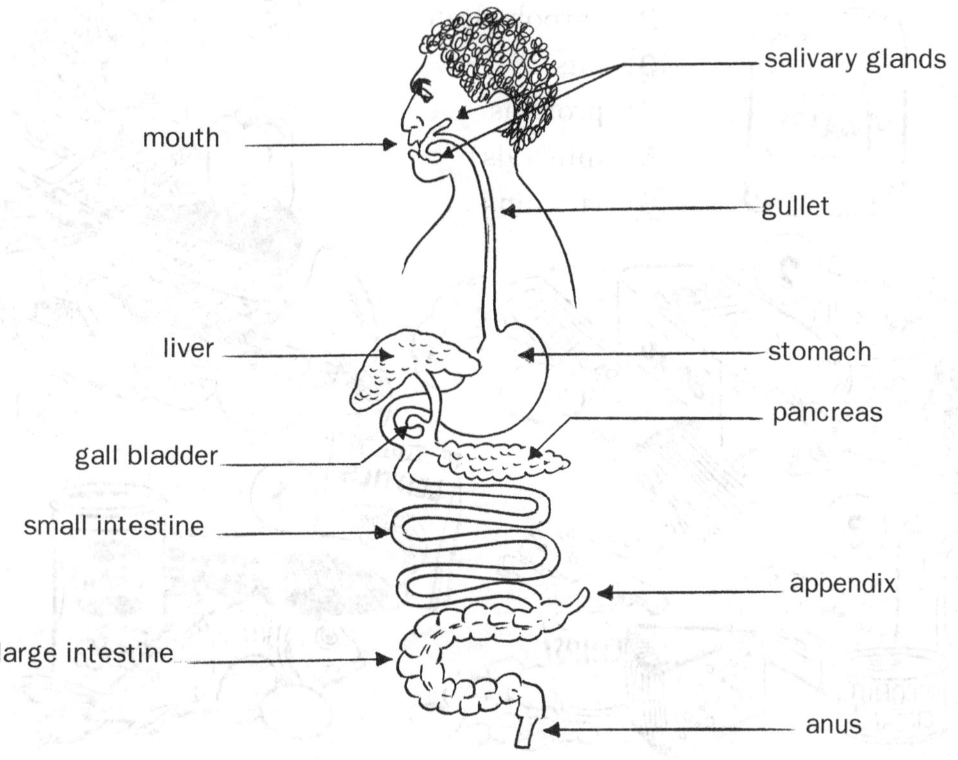

The blood distributes the nutrients to cells and tissues throughout the body. The body uses these nutrients for its own needs and functions. Most of the nutrients undergo chemical changes as they are used in the cells and tissues. These chemical changes produce waste products, which go into the bloodstream.

Some of the wastes are carried to the kidneys, which filter them from the blood. The body expels these wastes in the urine. The liver also filters out some wastes and concentrates them into a liquid called bile. Bile is stored in the gall bladder until it is needed to aid in digestion. Then the gall bladder empties bile into the small intestine. From there, any remaining bile passes into the large intestine, along with parts of the food not digested in the small intestine. The large intestine absorbs water and small amounts of minerals from this waste material. This material, along with bacteria present in the large intestine, becomes the final waste product, the faeces, and it is eliminated from the body.

 Kinds of nutrients

Nutritionists classify nutrients into six main groups:

1. water
2. carbohydrates
3. fats
4. proteins
5. minerals
6. vitamins

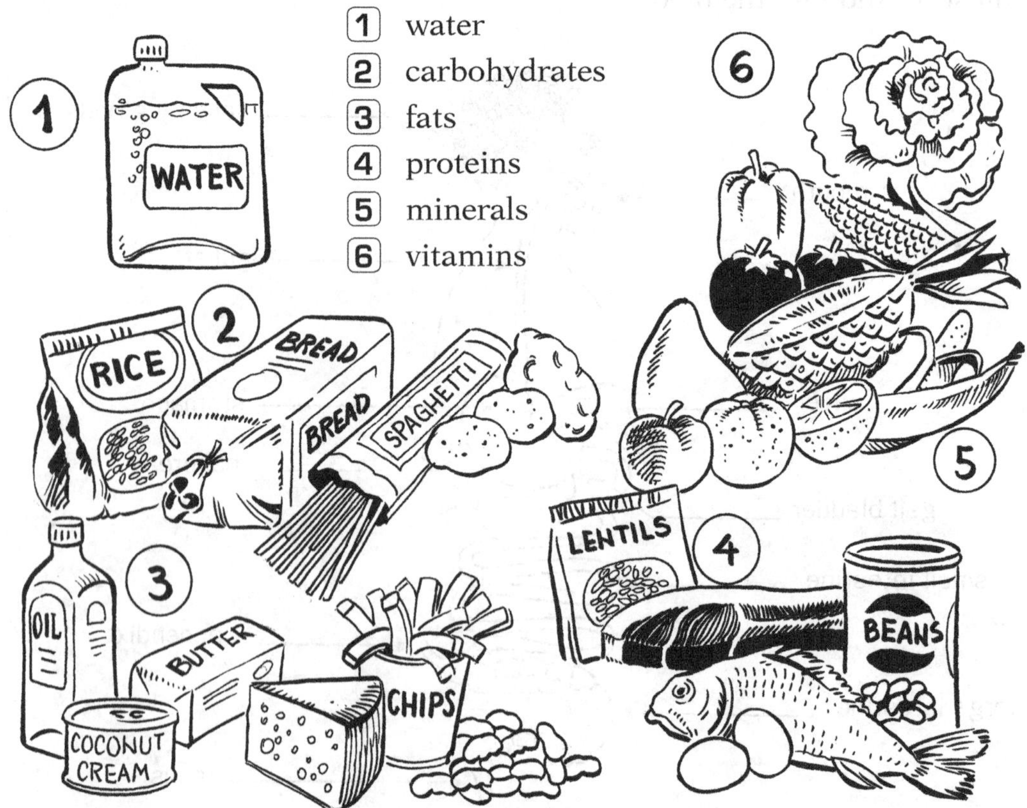

Water is needed in great amounts because the body consists largely of water. Usually, between 50 and 75 per cent of a person's body weight is made up of water.

The body requires large quantities of carbohydrates, fats and proteins because these nutrients provide energy.

Although minerals and vitamins are only needed in small amounts, they are as vital to health as any other nutrients. Minerals and vitamins are needed for growth and to maintain tissues and regulate body functions.

Water

Water is the most important nutrient as it helps dissolve other nutrients and transports them to all the tissues. The body can live without the other nutrients for several weeks but cannot do without water for more than a week. The chemical reactions that turn food into energy or tissue-building materials can take place only in a watery solution. The body also needs water to carry away waste products and to cool itself. Adults should have about 2.4 litres of water a day in the form of drinks or water in food.

Carbohydrates

The main source of energy for the body is carbohydrates. Most foods contain carbohydrates. Staple foods, such as sweet potato, cassava, cooking bananas, Singapore taro, taro, European potato, breadfruit, yam, sago, rice, kaukau, flour, bread and hard biscuits contain a large amount of carbohydrates. Other foods rich in carbohydrates include: beans, breads, cereals, corn, pasta (macaroni, spaghetti, and similar foods made of flour), peas and potatoes.

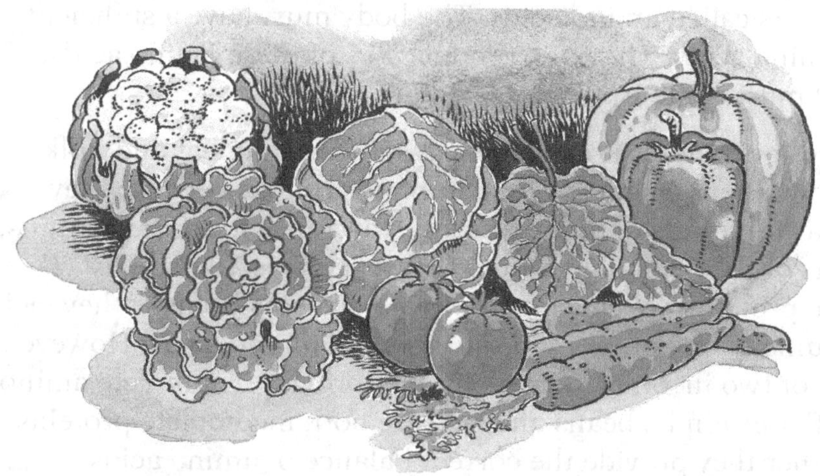

Fats

Fats are a highly concentrated source of energy. High energy foods are those that contain a large amount of fat or sugar. The main foods are cooking oils (like coconut, vegetable and palm oils), dripping, margarine, mature coconut cream, marita, peanut butter, pork fat, butter, packet sugar, sugar cane, jam and honey. Avocado, peanuts and other nuts also contain a lot of fat and can be included here, although they are listed in other food groups too.

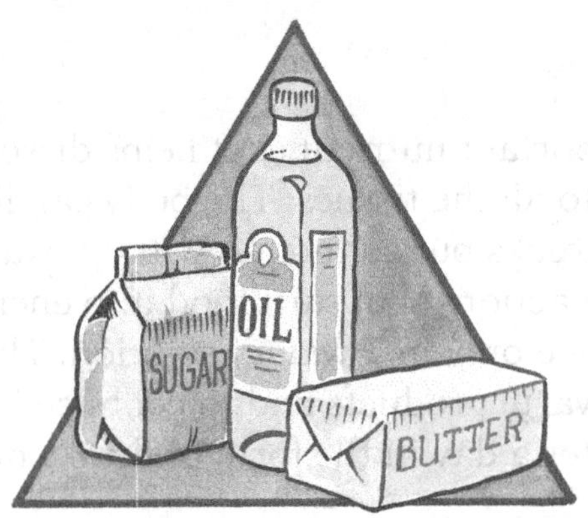

Proteins

Proteins provide energy like carbohydrates, but more importantly, proteins serve as one of the main building materials of the body. Muscle, skin, cartilage and hair, for example, are made up largely of proteins. In addition, every cell contains proteins called enzymes, which speed up chemical reactions. Cells could not function without these enzymes. Proteins also serve as hormones (chemical messengers) and as antibodies (disease-fighting chemicals). Proteins are large, complex molecules made up of smaller units called amino acids. The body must have a sufficient supply of 20 amino acids. The body produces 11 of these amino acids, but the other 9 must come from people's diets.

The best sources of proteins are cheese, eggs, fish, lean meat and milk. The proteins in these foods are called complete proteins because they contain adequate amounts of all the essential amino acids. Cereal grains, legumes (plants of the pea family), nuts and vegetables also supply proteins. These proteins are called incomplete proteins because they lack adequate amounts of one or more of the essential amino acids. However, a combination of two incomplete proteins can provide a complete amino acid mixture. For example, beans and rice are both incomplete proteins, but eaten together they provide the correct balance of amino acids.

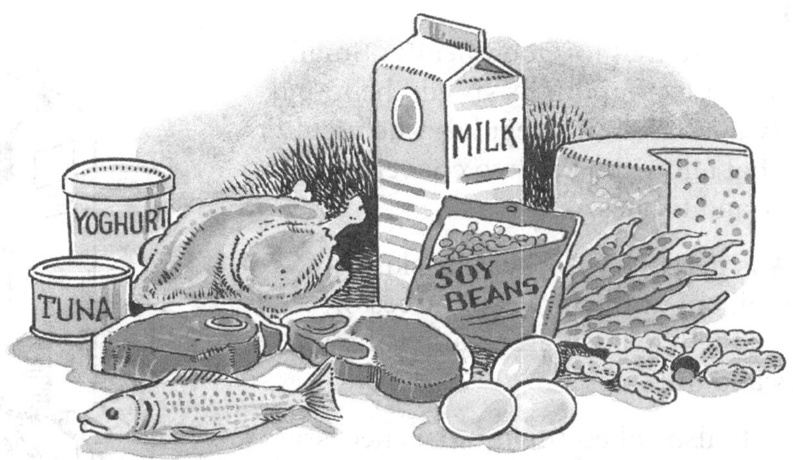

Minerals

Minerals are needed for the growth and maintenance of body structures. People only need small amounts of minerals each day.

Minerals are inorganic compounds, unlike vitamins, carbohydrates, fats and proteins. This means that they are not created by living things. Plants obtain minerals from the water or soil, and animals get minerals by eating plants or plant-eating animals. Unlike other nutrients, minerals are not broken down within the body.

The required minerals include calcium, chlorine, magnesium, phosphorus, potassium, sodium and sulphur. Calcium, magnesium and phosphorus are essential parts of the bones and teeth. In addition, calcium is necessary for blood clotting. Milk and milk products are the richest sources of calcium. Cereals and meats provide phosphorus. Whole-grain cereals, nuts, legumes and green leafy vegetables are good sources of magnesium.

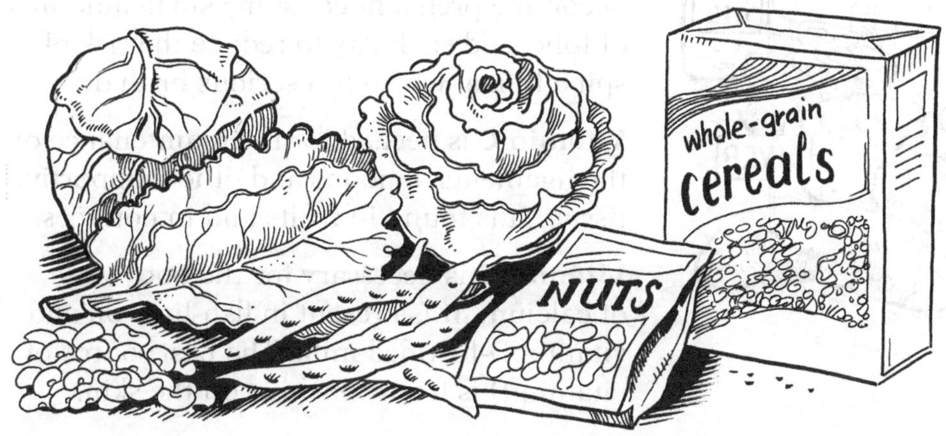

Vitamins

Vitamins are essential for good health. Small amounts of these compounds should be found in our daily diet. Vitamins regulate chemical reactions that allow the body to convert food into energy and tissues.

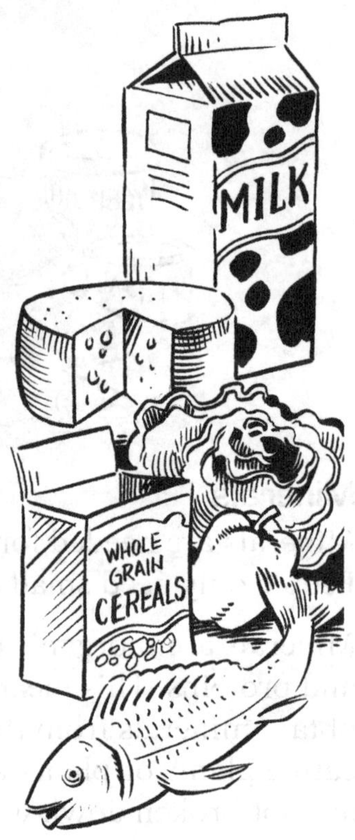

Vitamin A is necessary for healthy skin and development of the bones. Sources of this vitamin include liver, green and yellow vegetables and milk.

Vitamin B-1, also called thiamine, is necessary for changing starches and sugars into energy. It is found in meat and whole-grain cereals.

Vitamin B-2 is essential for complicated chemical reactions that take place during the body's use of food. Milk, cheese, fish, liver and green vegetables supply vitamin B-2.

Vitamin B-6 and two other B vitamins all play a role in chemical reactions essential for growth. Liver, yeast and many other foods contain these vitamins.

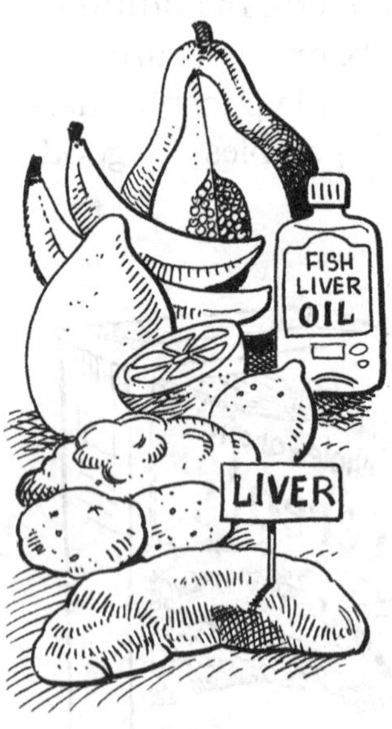

Vitamin B-12 and **folic acid** are both needed for forming red blood cells and for a healthy nervous system. Vitamin B-12 is found in animal products, especially liver. Folic acid is present in green leafy vegetables. Doctors recommend that all women who are capable of becoming pregnant consume small amounts of folic acid each day to reduce the risk of spina bifida, which is a serious birth defect.

Vitamin C is needed for the maintenance of the ligaments, tendons and other supportive tissue. It is found in fruits and in potatoes.

Vitamin D is necessary for the body's use of calcium. It is present in fish-liver oil and vitamin D-fortified milk. The best source of vitamin D is from sunshine on the skin.

Vitamin E helps maintain cell membranes. Vegetable oils and whole-grain cereals are especially rich in this vitamin. It is also found in small amounts in most meats, fruits and vegetables.

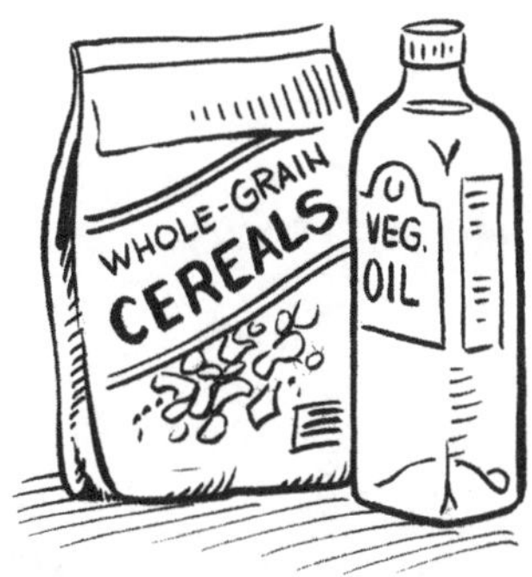

Vitamin K is necessary for proper clotting of the blood. Green leafy vegetables contain vitamin K. It is also manufactured by bacteria in the intestine.

INFORMATION

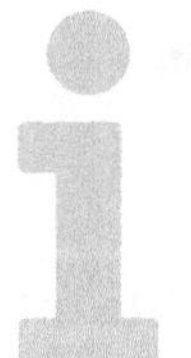

Some things you need to know!

→ Vitamin A deficiency

Do you know that people in the early stages of vitamin A deficiency normally have a condition called night blindness, which means they cannot see well in the dark? A healthy child has shiny, moist and smooth eyeballs while a child with severe vitamin A deficiency has dull, dry and rough eyes. This condition needs to be treated quickly. In the late stages of the disease, the eyeballs become soft and the surface of the eye breaks or bursts, causing permanent damage.

→ Prevention

The most effective preventive measure against vitamin A deficiency is a well-balanced diet. Eat brightly coloured vegetables and fruits, such as pumpkin, pawpaw and dark green leaves. Animal sources include eggs, liver, fish and milk. Vitamin A is a fat-soluble vitamin which can be stored in the body. Children who eat balanced diets based on a variety of foods should be safe from vitamin A deficiency.

 Guidelines for good nutrition

Eat a balanced diet. The key to good nutrition is a mixed diet that includes every kind of food group. To help in planning a balanced diet, nutritionists have devised systems that group foods according to nutrient content.

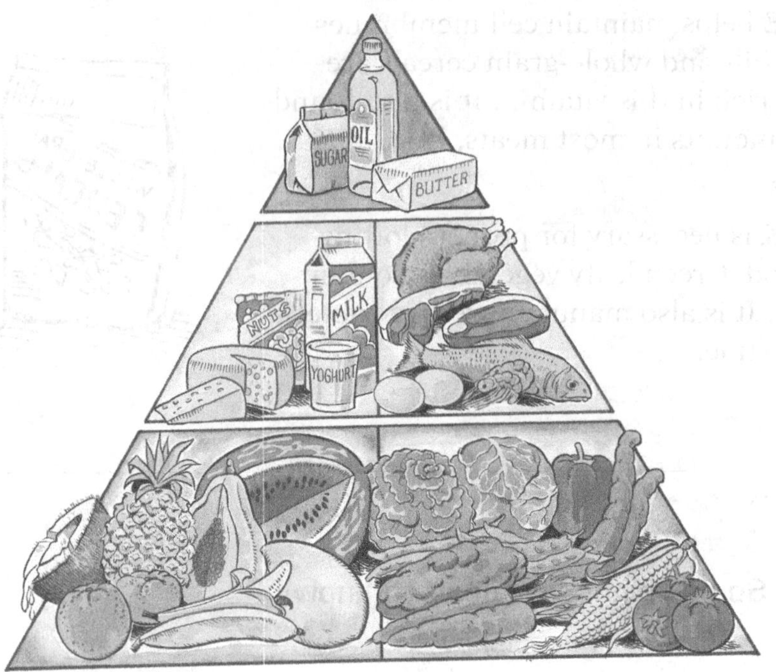

A People vary in their needs for energy. A person who plays sport daily, for example, needs more calories than someone who does little physical work. Children need enough calories to support their growth. Pregnant women need extra calories to provide enough nutrients for a healthy baby.

B Include fibre in your diet. Dietary fibre consists of complex carbohydrates that cannot be absorbed by the body. Fibre passes out of the body as waste. Fibre moves food along through the stomach and intestines, thus helping to prevent constipation (difficulty in emptying the intestine). Good sources of fibre include whole-grain breads and cereals, beans and peas, vegetables and fruit.

C Health experts recommend a diet that is low in saturated fats and cholesterol, which is a waxy substance found in many animal foods. Eating saturated fats and cholesterol raises the level of cholesterol in a person's blood. A high level of blood cholesterol increases the risk of heart disease. Animal products are the source of most saturated fats and all dietary cholesterol. To reduce the intake of saturated fats and cholesterol, health experts suggest choosing lean meats, fish, poultry with the skin removed, and low-fat dairy products. They also advise using fats and oils sparingly.

(D) Do not eat food with a lot of sodium and sugar. A diet that includes a great deal of sodium may increase the risk of high blood pressure. Sodium is found in many foods, including canned vegetables, frozen dinners, pickles, processed cheeses, table salt, and snack foods such as potato chips and nuts. One way to reduce sodium intake is to use herbs and other seasonings instead of salt in cooking and at the table. Another way is to select fresh foods rather than canned or frozen foods.

(E) Foods that contain a lot of sugar are often high in calories and fat but low in minerals, proteins and vitamins. Nutritionists sometimes call these foods 'empty calorie' foods, because they may make a person feel full but provide few nutrients. In addition, sugar that remains in and around the teeth contributes to tooth decay. Foods that have a large amount of sugar include lollies, pastries, many breakfast cereals, and sweetened canned fruits. In place of sugary foods, nutritionists advise people to snack on fresh fruits and vegetables. They also recommend that people drink unsweetened fruit and vegetable juices instead of soft drinks (a can of soft drink may contain 10 teaspoons of sugar or even more).

Food gives you energy to work and play. It is important to listen to your body's demands by eating the right amount and type of food so that it can function properly. This is especially important for children and teenagers because their bodies are still growing and need the right nutrients for growth to happen.

Eat enough food to keep to the right body weight. Your right weight is the weight that is best for the normal functioning of your body, based on your height and build. You look better and live longer if you are the right weight.

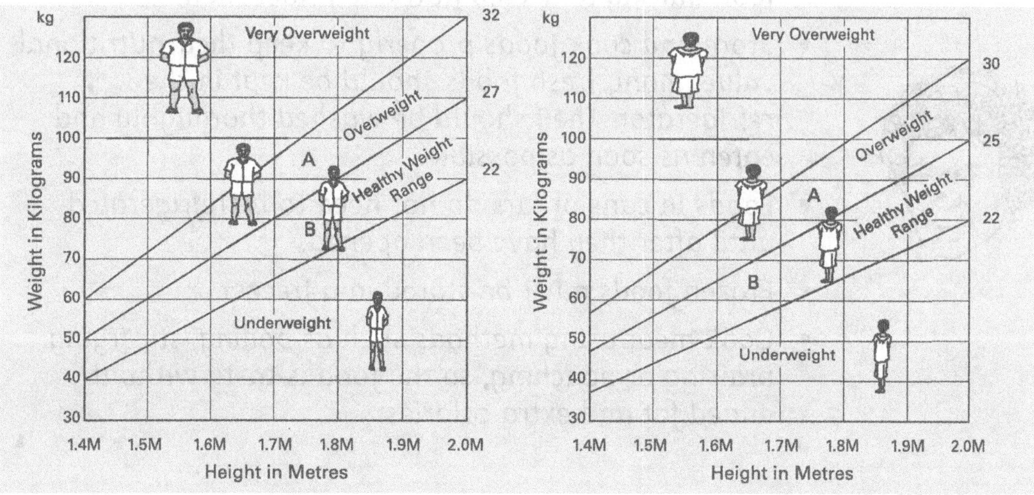

Try to follow these simple rules

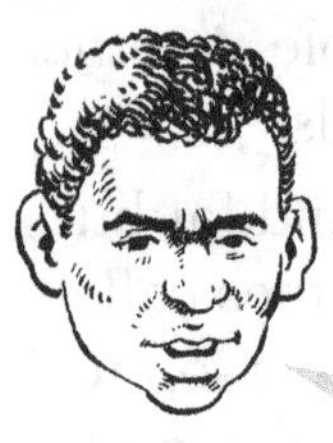

- Eat a variety of foods to give you a well-balanced diet. Eat the right kind of foods in the right amounts.
- Eat fish instead of meat and eat vegetables like beans and peas.
- Eat lots of fruit and vegetables. They will keep you healthy now and protect you against developing some diseases later in life.
- Avoid lollies and deep-fried fast foods.
- Consult a nutritionist on how to change your diet and exercise to be the right weight for your height.
- Exercise regularly, regardless of your weight.
- Weigh yourself from time to time to know if your weight is right.

Healthy tips

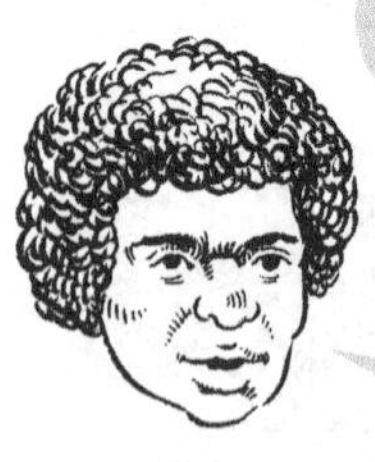

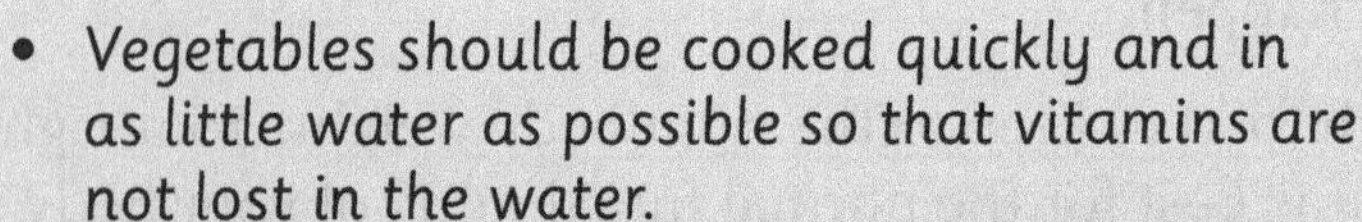

- Vegetables should be cooked quickly and in as little water as possible so that vitamins are not lost in the water.

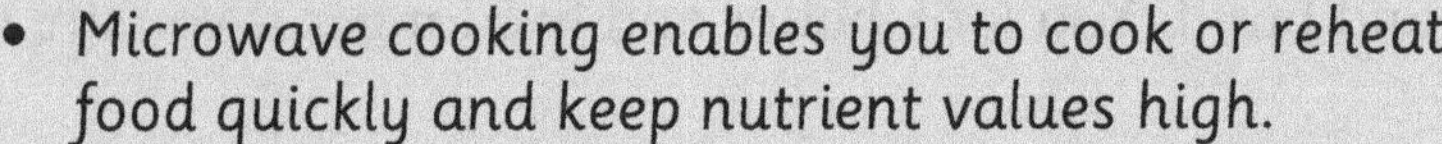

- Microwave cooking enables you to cook or reheat food quickly and keep nutrient values high.

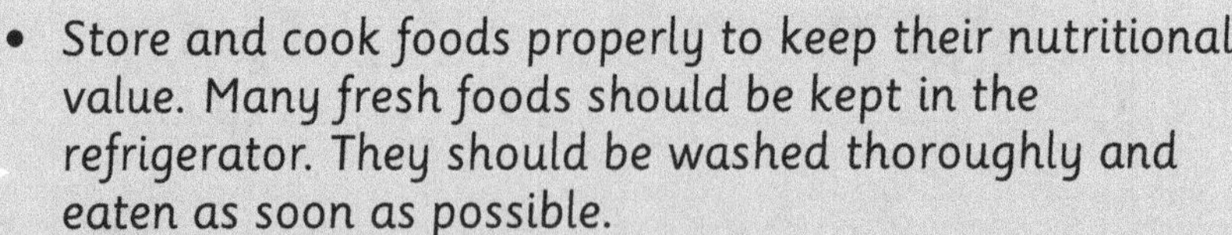

- Store and cook foods properly to keep their nutritional value. Many fresh foods should be kept in the refrigerator. They should be washed thoroughly and eaten as soon as possible.
- Foods in cans or jars do not need to be refrigerated until after they have been opened.
- Frozen foods must be stored in a freezer.
- Cook meat using methods such as boiling, stir-frying, braising or poaching, so the food is tasty without added fat and extra calories.

Be cautious about food myths and misinformation: ideas about foods may become popular, but they are not necessarily correct. For example, some people believe that if they take a vitamin pill every day they can eat whatever they choose. But in fact, people who rely on vitamin pills may not get the amount of calories, minerals or proteins that they need. Another common, but incorrect, idea is that such starchy foods as potatoes are fattening. In fact, starches provide fewer calories than do fats such as butter or margarine.

Dangers of an unhealthy lifestyle

The two biggest risks to someone's health are drinking too much alcohol and eating too much food.

Alcoholism

In PNG, alcohol is the cause of many incidents and problems. Many people think that alcohol is good for their health but in fact it is not.

Alcoholic drinks supply calories, but they provide almost no nutrients. In addition, alcohol is a powerful drug, and habitual drinking can lead to many health problems. Many people become addicted and cannot stop drinking alcohol until they are dead.

Health experts recommend that if people choose to drink alcoholic beverages, then they should consume only small amounts. They suggest that certain people avoid alcohol altogether: children and adolescents, pregnant women, people who are about to drive, anyone who is taking medicine, and those who are unable to limit their drinking.

Activity 1·1

Based on the above information, write an essay based on some of the experiences that you have seen in your family regarding alcohol.

Say whether alcohol is good for your health or not. Also include the advantages and the disadvantages alcohol has on the family.

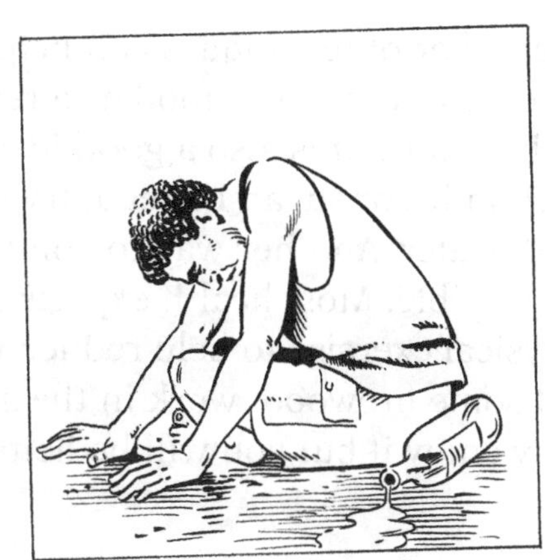

Obesity

Do not overeat. When a person gets more calories than are needed, the body stores most of the excess calories as fat. This can result in obesity. An obese person has too much body fat for good health. Obesity increases the risk of diseases such as adult-type diabetes, stroke, high blood pressure, gall bladder disease, heart disease and certain cancers. Health problems, such as osteoarthritis and lower back pain, are often worsened by the pressure of excess weight.

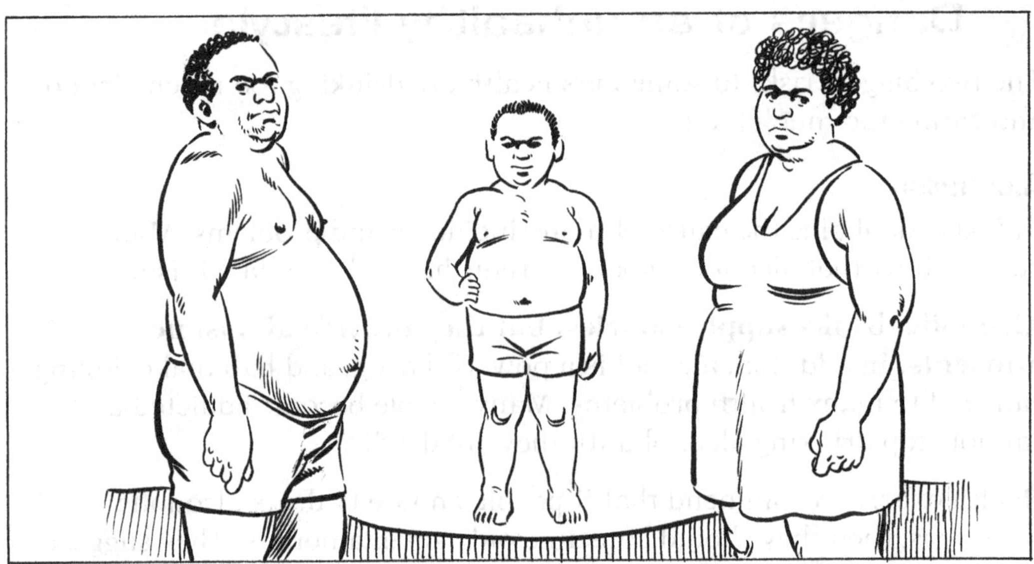

In many towns in Papua New Guinea the sale of lamb flaps is a popular treat. People love to buy the lamb flaps along with banana or sweet potatoes to supplement the other nutrients that the body needs.

Eating lamb flaps can gradually lead to obesity and can affect your health because they are very high in saturated fats.

A number of techniques can help a person avoid obesity. For one thing, be careful not to use food as a reward or as a way to overcome loneliness or boredom. It is also a good idea to avoid snacking on foods that are high in fat or sugar. Instead, try substituting fruits and fruit juice diluted with water. Another way to combat obesity is to be as physically active as possible. Most health experts recommend that a person engage in physical exercise to help reduce weight. Try to work around the house, cut some firewood, work in the garden or plant some seeds—you'll not only enjoy it but you will be helping your body get rid of excess fat.

Activity 1•2

In your free time, try to find out where people sell lamb flaps. Do some investigation to find out how much each piece costs compared to the actual price at the stores.

Find out how much money a person spends on buying lamb flaps compared to buying fresh healthy food from the market daily.

Analyse your findings and make a conclusion.

Discuss this issue with your friends and try to find a nutritionist who can help you answer some of your questions.

Agore's story

Agore sells food at the roadside. She makes around K30–K40 profit a day from her business. It is very profitable and she makes more money than her husband who works in a government office as a clerk.

'I sell cooked food at the offices and roadsides where there is a potential market,' she said.

'It is financially rewarding given the economic crisis that the country is facing.'

Agore is 34 years old and comes from Simbu province while her husband Tom is from Goroka. They have three children who go to school.

As for Tom, he says that Agore is a great help because she takes care of the food for the family on a daily basis as well as providing bus fares and lunch money for them all.

'I don't know what we would do without her. I guess I made the right choice in her,' he says proudly.

With unemployment rising, there are more women out there determined to bring back home something for the family to eat at the end of the day.

→

Asked what they thought of the situation, they raised their concerns saying that the government should help to educate them in how to handle food, to promote food hygiene, personal hygiene and basically health in general.

'Currently there is no effort from the Government to tackle the issue of unemployment so mothers are forced to go out and sell their food regardless of the safe health of the public at large,' said Agore.

'Sometimes the police and the securities come to our selling points and they kick our food and eskies saying that the sale of cooked food is illegal. We fight with them telling them that they are hypocrites and if we had our way, we would see to it that they are terribly punished,' she says.

Agore still sells her food to care for her family. Her husband Tom is working hard with the aim to invest some money to buy a better stove for her.

Activity 1·3

Based on Agore's Story, write a story about life in the city—think of some ways that you can help people to know more about food safety and health. Why is it important that the food sold is safe for people to eat?

Activity 1·4 *Healthy food*

Many products are advertised on television, radio and the newspapers by large commercial companies. These companies pay a lot of money to have their products advertised, for example beef biscuits, two-minute noodles, Ox and Palm, Diana Tuna and many other items too.

In this activity, you are asked to find out the following details:

- what foods are advertised?
- what claims are made about the foods?
- would you buy them as part of a healthy diet?
- how do you know if what the advertisement is saying is true?

Food advertised	What claims are made about the foods?	Would you buy this food as part of a healthy diet?	How do you know if what the advertisement is saying is true?	Name of TV station	Other medium

Compare your answers with your friends in class and write a report titled, 'The Media and Nutrition in Papua New Guinea'.

Chapter 2 Nutrition and disease

An improper or inadequate diet can lead to a number of diseases—good nutritional habits can help prevent certain diseases.

Heart disease

Heart disease in its most common form is called coronary artery disease (CAD). CAD narrows the coronary arteries and so reduces the blood supply to the heart. It can lead to severe attacks of chest pain and, eventually, to life-threatening heart attacks. High blood pressure and high levels of blood cholesterol are two of the major risk factors for CAD. High blood pressure and high levels of blood cholesterol can often be lessened by having a healthy diet.

Many people with mild high blood pressure can reduce it by limiting their intake of salt and calories. Similarly, many people can lower their blood cholesterol level by reducing the amount of fat (particularly saturated fat), cholesterol and calories in their diet. They can do this by avoiding foods such as butter, cakes, cookies, egg yolks, fatty meats, tropical oils and whole-fat dairy products.

Cancer

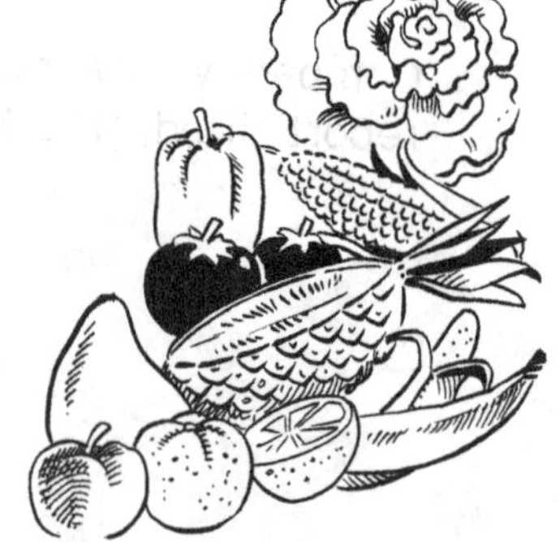

Scientists do not know exactly why cancer develops, but they have found that heredity, environment and lifestyle all play a role in causing the disease. They have also learned that good nutrition can help prevent certain kinds of cancer in laboratory animals. Large doses of vitamins A and C have been proved to prevent some cancers in animals. Many scientists believe that certain foods contain substances that may help prevent some cancers in people. Such foods include broccoli, cabbage, carrots, cauliflower, fruits, spinach, whole-grain breads and cereals, and some seafood. Lessening the intake of fats and increasing the intake of fibre may also help prevent some cancers from forming.

Deficiency diseases

Many diseases result from the deficiency (lack) of certain nutrients in the diet. When the missing nutrient is provided, the disease usually can be eliminated. Deficiency diseases are most widespread in developing countries, where people often lack access to adequate food supplies.

Protein-energy malnutrition

Protein-energy malnutrition (PEM), also called protein calorie malnutrition, occurs when the diet is low in both proteins and calories. If the diet is especially low in proteins, the condition is called kwashiorkor. Signs of kwashiorkor include changes in the colour and texture of the hair and skin, swelling of the body, and damage to the intestines, liver and pancreas. The disease usually attacks children who are suffering from an infectious disease. Kwashiorkor is fatal unless the patient is given protein along with food to provide calories. If the diet is especially low in calories, the condition is called marasmus. Marasmus usually attacks infants and young children, and it causes extreme underweight and weakness.

Protein-energy malnutrition is a common problem in Papua New Guinea. It is caused by not eating enough energy foods and sometimes not enough protein providing foods.

Activity 2·1

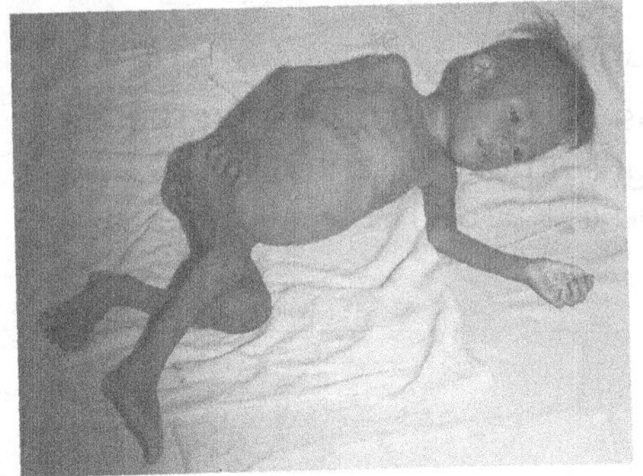

Look at the picture of someone with PEM and discuss how this deficiency is caused and how to prevent it.

Visit a hospital and meet some children and adults with PEM. Write a report after your visit. What have you found out?

According to health workers, young children are the most affected group. At birth, these children are small in weight and already growth-stunted. They will be small for their age, unlike normal babies who look healthy and strong.

Health experts have said that there are other ways to treat PEM. Because a child's weight can drop quickly, treatment begins at the outpatient clinics as soon as a child's weight has stopped increasing.

The health worker or nurse will treat the child and give advice on further treatment.

Activity 2·2

Using information from health workers, design a diet for PEM sufferers using food readily available, such as fish from the market, greens, sweet potatoes, and fresh fruit like guava, pawpaw or orange.

Write up this diet as a poster and include pictures of essential foods. Display this poster in community or health centres as well as on school notice boards.

However, if there is no improvement in the child, then the child is admitted to hospital where the health extension officer, sister and the nutrition staff will make sure that proper treatment is given for the child to recover.

INFORMATION

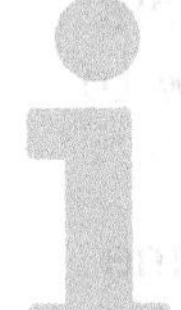

Important points to remember

Protein-energy malnutrition is caused by not eating the right kinds of foods in the right amounts, and it is the most common form of malnutrition in Papua New Guinea.

Activity 2·3

Do a mini survey in your community about protein-energy malnutrition. Ask your parents to help you if possible.

Questionnaire

Name: ____

Age: ______ Gender: ____________ Marital status: ____________

Question 1: What is protein-energy malnutrition (PEM)? __________

____

____

____

Question 2: How can you treat a PEM patient? ______________

____

____

____

Question 3: What do you know about diarrhoea?

____

____

____

Question 4: Can diarrhoea be treated? Explain how.

____

____

____

Question 5: How can one identify a person with vitamin A deficiency?

____

____

____

Note: Select only five people to interview and present your findings to your parents for discussion.

Bring the findings back to your school and compare your answers with your classmates.

The teacher can assist you by organising a debate about it.

Vitamin deficiencies

The signs and symptoms of vitamin deficiencies vary according to the missing vitamin. Vitamin C deficiency, also called scurvy, causes sore and bleeding gums, slow repair of wounds and painful joints. Vitamin D deficiency, also called rickets, causes an abnormal development of the bones.

Mineral deficiencies

The most common mineral deficiency disease is iron-deficiency anaemia, which results from a lack of iron. In a person with this disease, the blood does not have enough healthy red blood cells and cannot supply the tissues with sufficient oxygen. Thus, the person feels weak or tired. Other symptoms include dizziness, headaches, rapid heartbeat, and shortness of breath.

Other diseases

Other diseases may result from poor nutritional habits. For example, the excessive intake of alcohol causes some forms of liver disease. Obesity increases the risk of gall bladder disease and diabetes in adults. The risk of osteoporosis (loss of bone tissue) is higher for women, especially if their intake of calcium and level of physical activity are low. To prevent osteoporosis, physicians recommend a lifelong combination of regular exercise and a diet with adequate calcium.

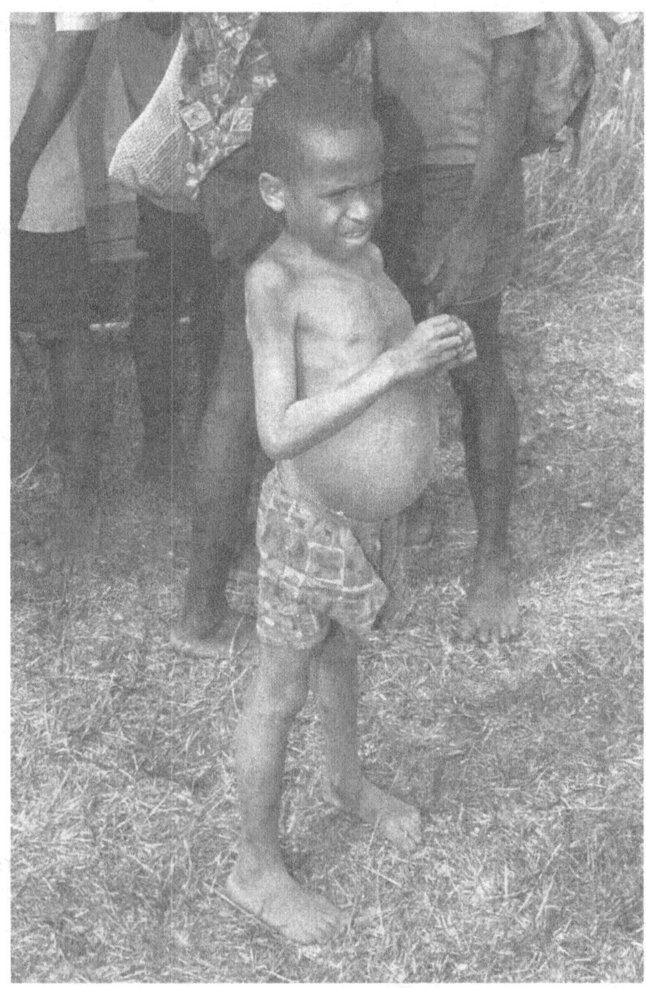

Activity 2·4

Check your knowledge by answering the following questions:

1. Why is water an essential nutrient?
2. How do complete proteins differ from incomplete proteins?
3. What are some foods that supply complete proteins?
4. What are some symptoms of iron-deficiency anaemia?
5. Why must essential fatty acids be included in the diet?
6. What is kwashiorkor? What is marasmus?
7. What are the dangers of obesity?
8. What are some ways to reduce sodium intake?
9. What are the three main functions of nutrients in the body?
10. Why is it important to include fibre in the diet?

Chapter 3 Importance of hygiene

What is hygiene?

Hygiene 'is the things that people do in order to stay healthy, like washing regularly, having clean water, clean toilets and clean kitchen, proper rubbish disposal, keeping food covered or in the refrigerator.'

K. Rouse, *Health for the Pacific A–Z of Essential Terms*, page 66.

Why is hygiene important?

Hygiene is important because it helps to keep everyone healthy. Poor hygiene conditions in the home environment lead to disease and illness. We also need to ensure that we keep our body clean—good personal hygiene is as important as good hygiene conditions in our home environment.

Personal hygiene is essential for all people so that they have a healthy lifestyle. People need:

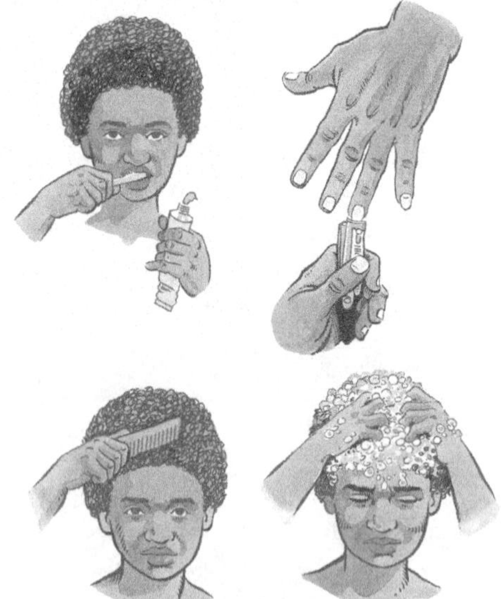

- ☑ to have plenty of water for washing purposes
- ☑ to develop good habits of personal hygiene and cleanliness, such as washing their bodies and hair regularly, washing hands before handling and eating food, keeping nails short so that germs do not spread, cleaning teeth to prevent bad breath and gum disease and use clean toilet habits
- ☑ to get rid of body waste by going to a toilet or in a hole away from the house, or covering faeces with soil. It must be kept away from any water supply.

Hygiene around the home environment goes hand in hand with personal hygiene. People need:

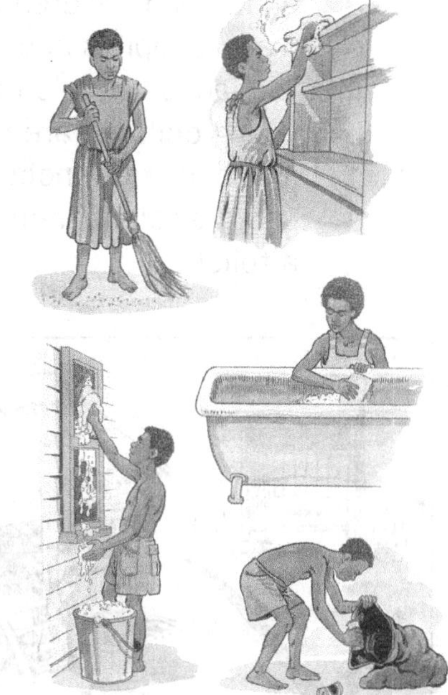

- to keep their living conditions clean and free of pests that can spread disease
- to have neat and tidy houses,
- to have a clean yard with proper drainage to prevent mosquitoes from breeding in water
- to have clean clothing
- to use plant waste as compost
- to bury other rubbish away from the house and drinking water supply
- to keep toilet facilities away from the house and water supply.

What are some effects of poor hygiene?

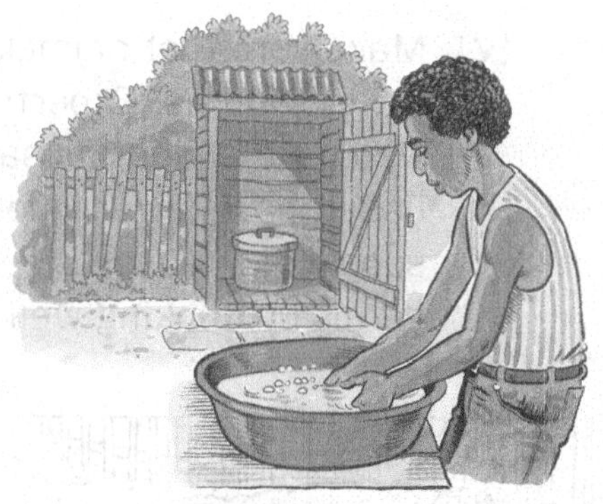

- People forget to wash their hands and faces without knowing that germs and dirt can make them very sick. Washing your face and hands with soap means eating clean food without germs. Soap must be available every time you need to wash your face and hands. Remember to wash your hands after coming from the toilet, and also after cleaning a child's bottom after defecating. After gardening, wash hands with soap and water. Wash a child's hands before meals because children have a habit of sucking their fingers.
- It is a health issue for families to have a clean toilet. Diarrhoea comes from germs found in human faeces. Germs can get into your body through drinking dirty water. Germs can get onto food, onto hands, or onto utensils and surfaces used for preparing food.

To prevent this happening, use a toilet. Where there are no toilets, adults and children must defecate well away from houses, paths, water supplies and anywhere that children play. After defecating, the faeces should be buried. It is said that faeces of babies and young children are even more infectious than those of adults. So it is better to encourage children to use toilets. If children do not use the toilet, then it is healthy to bury the faeces or put it down a toilet.

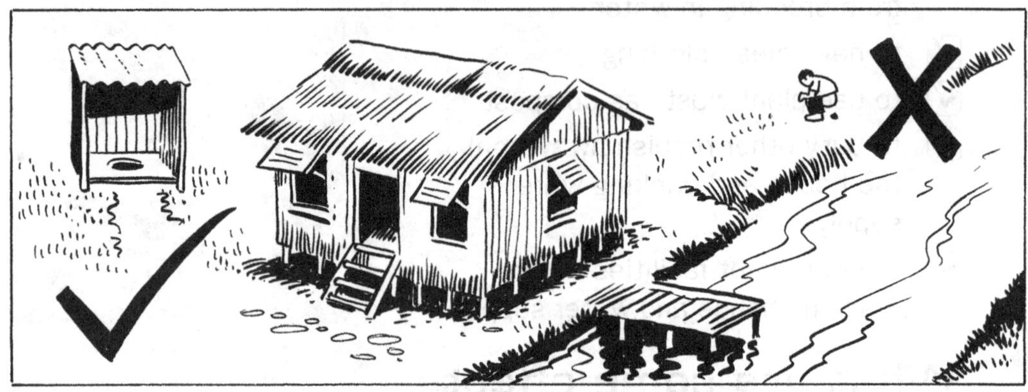

☑ Make sure that animals' faeces are kept away from homes and water sources. Experts in environmental health say that families who have a plentiful safe piped water supply and know how to use it, have fewer illnesses. Families without a safe piped water supply can reduce illness if they protect their water supply from germs by drinking well water that is far away from a toilet.

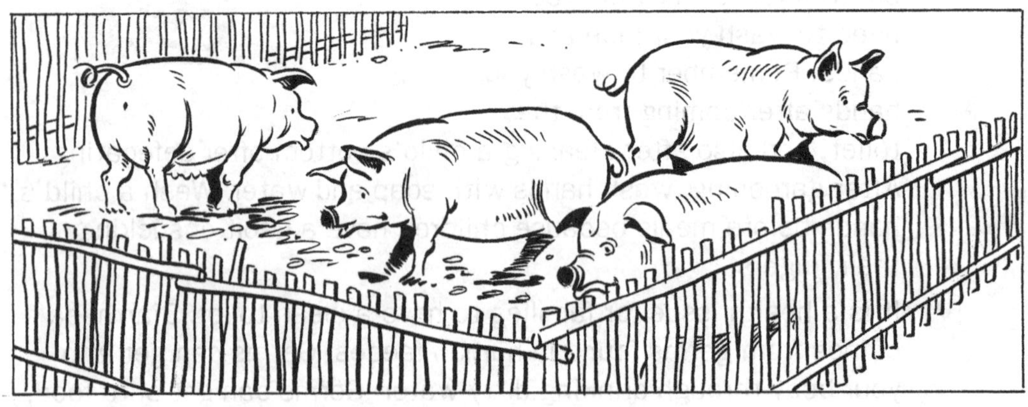

Drinking water must be covered properly to keep germs away. Buckets, ropes, water bottles and containers used to collect and store water must be kept as clean as possible. Keep animals away from drinking water. Take water out of a container with a clean cup. Do not drink water with dirty hands. Keep animals out of the house.

- ☑ Clean water does not mean that it is germ free. The safest drinking water is from a piped supply or from an underground spring. Water from other sources is likely to contain germs. Water drawn from sources such as ponds, streams, wells, tanks or public stand pipes should be boiled and then cooled before drinking. Boiling drinking water kills germs fast. After it cools down, it is safe to give to young children for drinking.

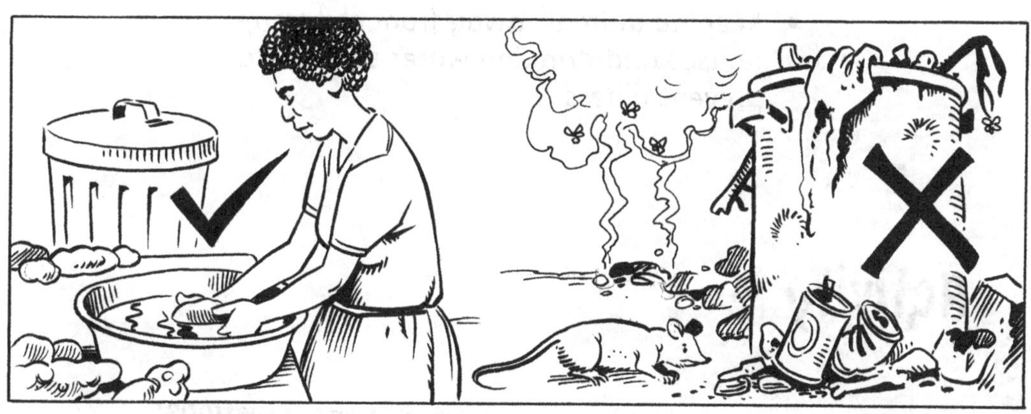

- ☑ Eating contaminated food causes illness. To avoid being ill, make sure that food is thoroughly cooked, especially meat, fish and chicken. Eat food soon after it has cooked, so that it does not turn bad. If food has to be kept for more than five hours, it should either be kept heated or kept cooled.
- ☑ Keep food clean and covered away from flies, cockroaches, rats, mice and other animals. Germs breed in rubbish, such as scraps and peelings from fruit and vegetables. Every family should have a special pit where household rubbish is buried or burned everyday.
- ☑ Do not let animals lick children's hands and faces. Pets must be well fed and clean. Keep animals, such as pigs, well away from living quarters. Wash hands with soap and water after handling animals and their faeces.

Key pointers

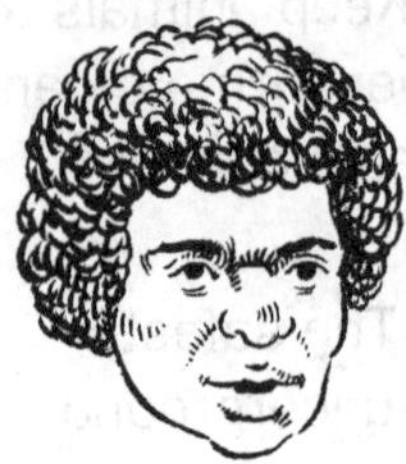

- Using proper toilets can prevent illness.
- Burning or burying household rubbish can prevent illness.
- Keeping food in a safe and clean place can prevent illness.

- Using clean safe healthy water can prevent illness.
- Boiling drinking water can prevent illness.
- Keeping animals away from children, houses and drinking water sources can prevent illness.

Activity 3·1

Check your knowledge by answering these questions:

1 What do you know about food hygiene?
2 Do you think that sleeping with pigs and dogs in the house is hygienic?
3 Why should pit toilets be built far from water wells?
4 How do flies contaminate drinking water and food for eating?
5 Write a short report on the hygiene practices of your local community.

Chapter 4 Why we need safe drinking water

A clean, convenient water supply is necessary for people's health and hygiene.

- ☑ Dirty drinking water can carry diseases.
- ☑ People need enough water to keep themselves clean, because if the body is not washed regularly then skin infections and other diseases will occur.

Scarcity of water becomes an issue when there is no rain or where there is a lack of water in communities and villages.

In many places, water is piped and filtered straight to the homes for use. However in other places, water is not filtered but is still piped straight to the home for use. This is dangerous as the water may be contaminated and may cause sickness and death. The Secretary of Health, Dr Mann, states that the aim of the National Department of Health is to achieve maximum coverage for safe water in the country. He admits that it is difficult to identify problem areas in rural places unlike the city where we know where the water is piped to various communities. He points out that rural communities need to take a serious look at this safe water issue. Rural people need to fence their domesticated animals so that they do not defecate in the streams and pollute the waterways, and cemeteries and toilets should not be close to rivers or wells as this causes health risks.

 Why safe drinking water is needed

In Papua New Guinea people get their water from streams, rivers (surface water) and wells (ground water) or collect rain water in containers. In the larger urban centres, houses are connected to piped water from dams.

To have a clean water supply, water must be kept free of body and food waste because:

- ☑ contaminated water will cause water-borne disease in people as this water contains foreign substances such as chemicals that affect the quality of water
- ☑ most water-borne disease occurs from contaminated food and water
- ☑ drinking contaminated water will result in diseases such as gastroenteritis, typhoid, dysentery, cholera and infectious hepatitis.

Guidelines for ensuring a healthy water supply

- *Water must be boiled before drinking unless it comes from a chlorinated town supply or is guaranteed to be clean by the authorities.*
- *Water should be boiled for two minutes from the time it starts to boil.*
- *Water left to cool should be properly covered to avoid contamination.*

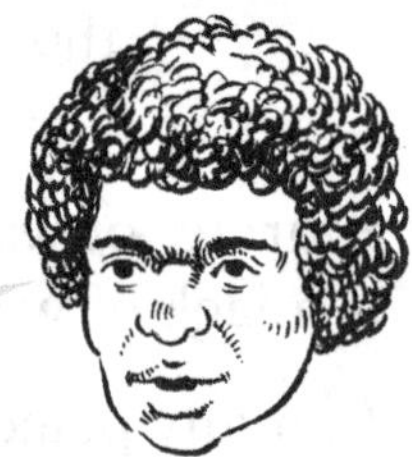

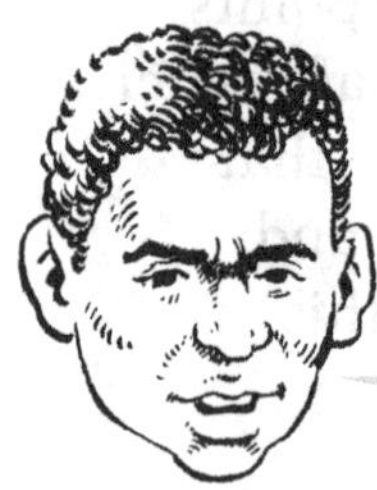

- *Water must be treated for human consumption—free from germs and bacteria that may be harmful to the community.*
- *Tank water must be filtered and treated with chlorine before consumption. It must have the first flush system so that debris from the roof does not go into the tank.*
- *Avoid defecating into a water source. Keep pets and animals away from water sources as they will contaminate the water.*
- *All broken water pipes, leakages from toilets or tanks must be reported to the authorities to take action.*

A common situation in Papua New Guinea

'People selling iced water in public should be taught basic healthy rules before selling it to the public for consumption,' said Dr Nicholas Mann, Secretary for Health. 'Scarcity of water especially during the dry period is obvious but nevertheless safe and clean healthy drinking water is important for everyone,' he said.

Papua New Guineans need to earn money and water business is part of survival. Dr Mann states that little business ventures, like selling iced water, should not be discouraged, but people need to be educated to sell safe iced water as a lot of iced water sold currently is unsafe water. Dr Mann states that:

- ☑ water must be boiled to get rid of any bacteria that cause diarrhoea and other water-borne diseases
- ☑ storing water in cordial containers is not safe because a temperature change can cause the plastic to become toxic and to contaminate the water. People need to use water containers that are resistant to temperature change, such as glass and metal containers
- ☑ people selling water who have diarrhoea, flu or other sicknesses, should not handle water, because they may transmit the virus to the consumer
- ☑ parents and teachers have a duty to teach their children about safe clean and healthy drinking water
- ☑ children must have their own water bottles and should not drink a lot of cordial or fruit juice. They should have natural water for lunch, which is healthy.

Although the sale of iced water is a concern, there is no clear evidence that it has caused a health problem or is the cause of an epidemic. However, it is important that the people who are selling iced water for public consumption sell safe water. They must understand why safe and clean drinking water is important for all people's health.

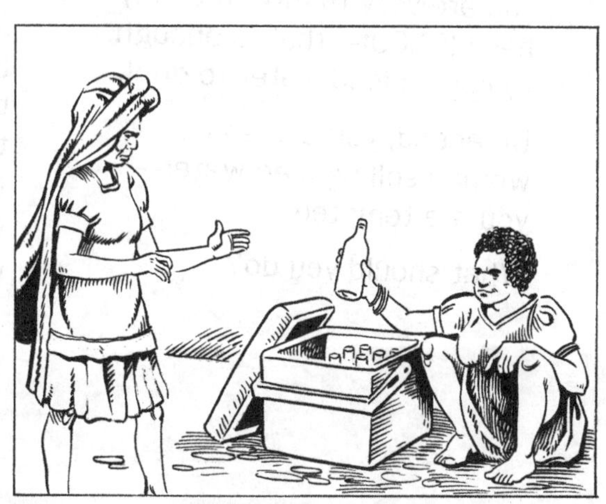

Healthy tips

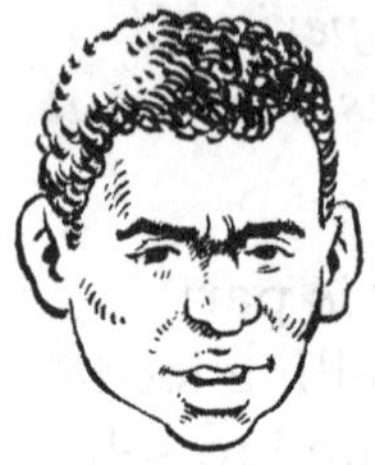

- *Wash your hands before handling and storing water containers.*
- *Wash containers thoroughly before storing water.*
- *Make sure that all containers have lids to avoid contamination from flies and other insects.*

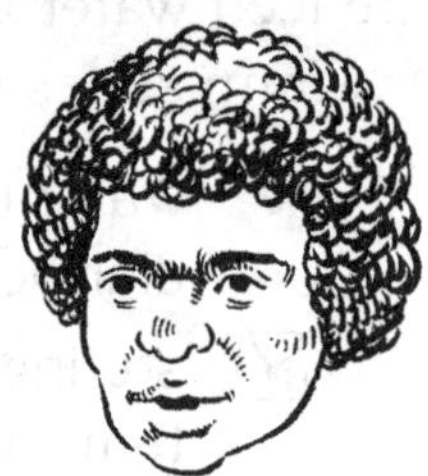

- *Boil water and refrigerate before drinking.*
- *Remember that safe and clean drinking water is good for your health.*

Activity 4·1

Situation 1

The sun is shining, the temperature is 38 degrees and you are very thirsty. You only have K0.60t—that is enough to buy an iced water to drink.

Up ahead, you see some women selling iced water—you are tempted.

What should you do?

Situation 2

You have gone home for your holidays and you notice that your family members have decided to build the toilet near the river. They say that it is better because after using the toilet, you can walk to the river to wash and fetch water for drinking and cooking.

What is your response to this situation?

What can you do to educate them about the danger?

Chapter 5 How to plan for a healthy lifestyle

What we need for a healthy lifestyle

A healthy lifestyle means that everyone must:

- ☑ live in a clean environment
- ☑ have a healthy diet
- ☑ have good personal hygiene.

Towards a clean home environment

To plan a healthy lifestyle everyone needs to live in a clean environment. This means that:

- ☑ the house needs to be well maintained, clean and free of pests
- ☑ the house must be an adequate size for the number of people living there
- ☑ the house must be free of rubbish—rubbish can be buried if it cannot be recycled
- ☑ there is good land drainage to prevent mosquitoes from breeding
- ☑ there is a good supply of clean water
- ☑ people are able to dispose of rubbish correctly.

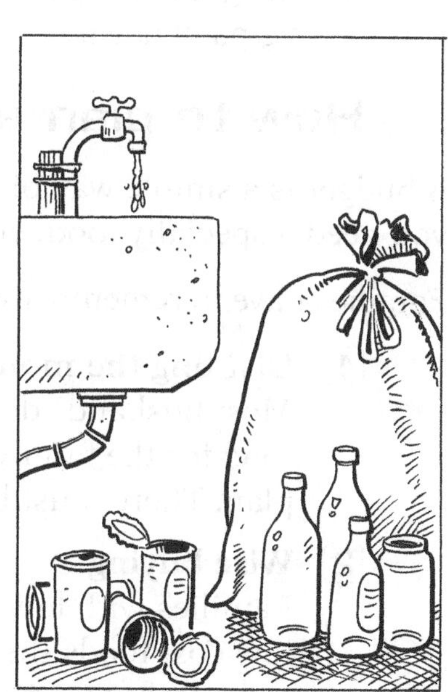

Rubbish must always be buried, placed in covered containers, burnt or taken away, because it attracts flies, pests and insects to breed in it. This can bring sicknesses to you and your family. Protect yourself from illnesses by being careful with your rubbish.

There are different types of rubbish. Some are useful for the garden, for example vegetable peelings.

- ☑ Place rubbish in covered containers or bags and ask your parents to have them ready for disposal.
- ☑ Set aside empty cans and bottles and sell them for recycling.
- ☑ Keep rivers, lakes, beaches and other public places clean from rubbish. Help your community to keep the surroundings, clean.
- ☑ Look after your plants and gardens well and keep them clean.
- ☑ Keep the parks, market places and bus stops clean.
- ☑ Keep your rubbish in a bag until you get home and dispose of it properly.

Towards a healthy diet

To plan a healthy diet everyone needs to:

- ☑ plan meals so that the 'right' foods are eaten. This means that the meals have food from all food groups (which includes water)
- ☑ plan gardens so that the 'right' foods can be grown
- ☑ budget family money so that the foods that cannot be grown can be purchased.

How to plan a budget

A budget is a simple way of planning how to spend your money on things you need, especially food, clothes, water, school fees and so on.

Families have to remember many things when planning their food budgets.

1. **Dividing the money**
   Most husbands do not give enough money to their wives to buy food for the family. Parents need to be firm with their budget plan. There must be some money put aside for food.
2. **Wise buying**
   Families with low incomes must choose the most nutritious low-cost foods they can find. Junk food from canteens, such as lamb flaps, fried flour and other foods, are bad for people's health. Compare prices of goods at different shops in order to get the most reasonably priced item. This may be time-consuming but it is worth the effort.

③ **Storage**

Think of where to store your food so that it is not spoilt by pests or insects before it is eaten. Some fresh foods, such as green leaves, should be bought daily. Tinned foods, such as tinned fish or meat, should be eaten as soon as they are opened. However, dried beans and peanuts keep for a very long time if they are stored in a cool, dry place. It is useful to have some dried vegetable proteins on hand for times when other protein foods may be unavailable.

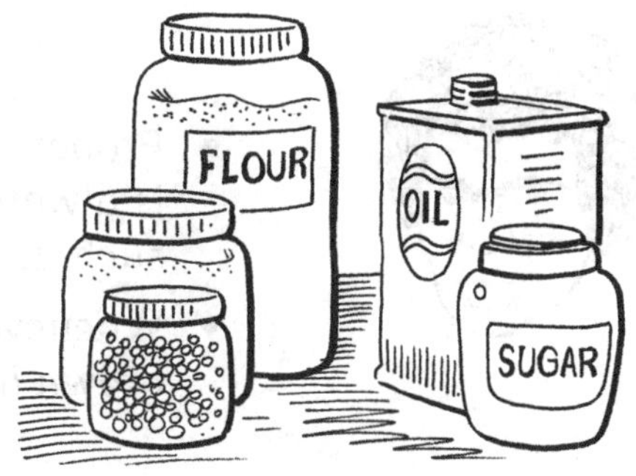

④ **Gardening**

Families with any land at all, whether they live in the city or village, must have a garden. They can grow most of the food they need, and always have a fresh supply on hand. It is more cost effective to grow your own food than to buy it elsewhere.

⑤ **Selling wisely**

Many families like to sell most of their good food and keep the less nutritious food for themselves, such as pale green cabbages, cucumbers and others. It is far better to grow good food, such as vegetables, and keep enough supplies for your family with some to sell to buy basic things like kerosene, flour, rice, batteries, oil, matches and other items.

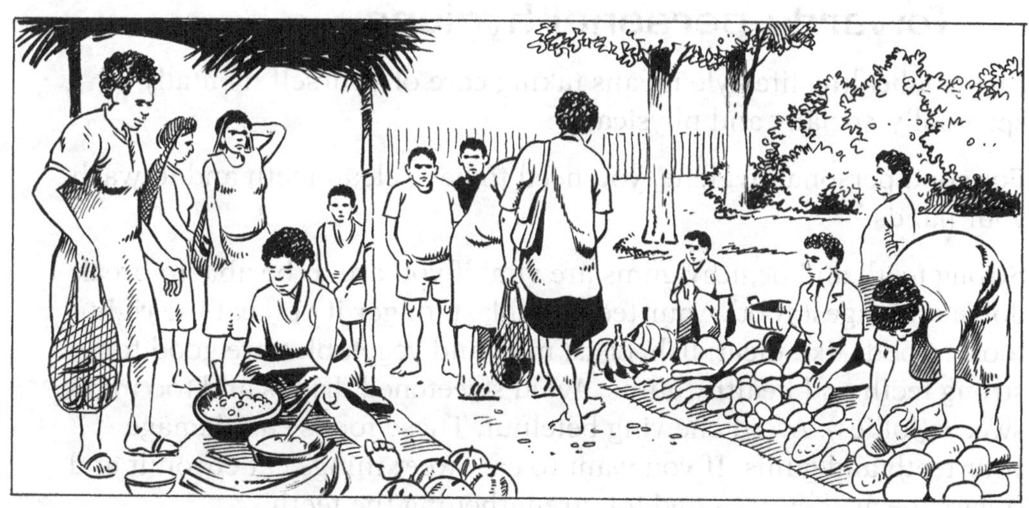

Important points to remember

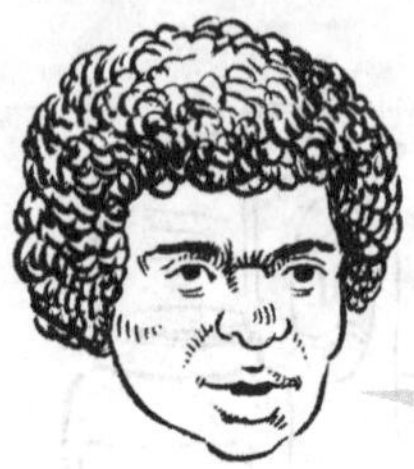

- Proper budgeting is essential to ensure that there is always enough money for all the necessities, such as food, school fees and emergencies.
- Whenever possible, nutritious foods should be grown in the family garden for home eating.

To make a food budget, a family needs to know:

- how much food each member of the family requires each day
- the total food required by the family
- the cost of the foods eaten by the family.

- Money should not be wasted on non-nutritious foods or unhealthy activities, such as gambling or drinking alcohol.
- Families should remember to buy food from the least expensive shops.

Towards personal hygiene

Living a healthy lifestyle means taking care of yourself mentally, spiritually, socially and physically.

For good personal hygiene, you need to have clean teeth and to wash your hands.

Strong teeth and healthy gums are vital if you are to be able to break down and digest food. Your teeth will last longer if you eat the right foods. Foods like meat, fish, eggs, milk and vegetables are good for strong teeth and healthy gums. Avoid sweetened drinks and too many sweets (lollies). Avoid chewing betelnut. These foods can damage your teeth and gums. If you want to eat sweet things eat coconut and sugarcane as they are good for strengthening the teeth.

Don't forget:

- ☑ to clean your teeth after breakfast, after lunch, and after dinner. Use a toothpick or dental floss. Germs live on dirty teeth—don't give them any chance to start holes
- ☑ that a fresh breath means a clean mouth and teeth
- ☑ to visit a dentist at least once a year to check if your teeth have any cavities
- ☑ that if you do not have a toothbrush, you can clean your teeth with a piece of twig or betelnut skin.

Wash hands before eating

Germs are microscopic and live in dirty places where you cannot see them. They can make you very sick. You can catch germs by eating food with dirty hands. Wash your hands thoroughly with soap and water. It is all right if you do not have soap, but wash your hands properly and rinse off with clean water. Keep your fingernails short because it prevents germs from settling under the nails and contaminating the food you eat.

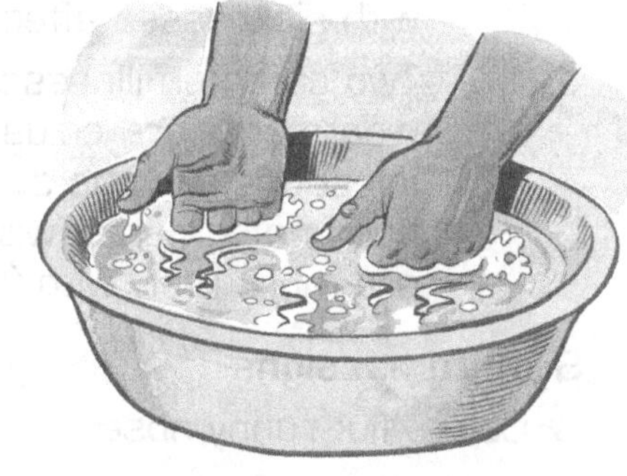

Remember to wash your hands:

- ☑ before eating or touching food
- ☑ after using the toilet
- ☑ after playing.

Wash wounds with soap and water

Always wash wounds to keep them clean and free of infection. A wound is an open cut—small, big or deep. A wound can sometimes have blood coming from it or a little or no blood at all. This can be a bruise but nevertheless keep the bruise clean and dry so it can heal quickly. Keep wounds covered.

Remember:

- ☑ wash wounds with soap and water—if possible with cooled boiled water
- ☑ ensure you receive antibiotics from your doctor or health centre if the wound becomes red or swollen, has pus (yellowish fluid coming out of it) and gives you pain.

For burn wounds, it is advisable to pour cold water on the burn or place it in cold water for at least five minutes. Remember that a hospital or health centre can help you if you burn yourself badly.

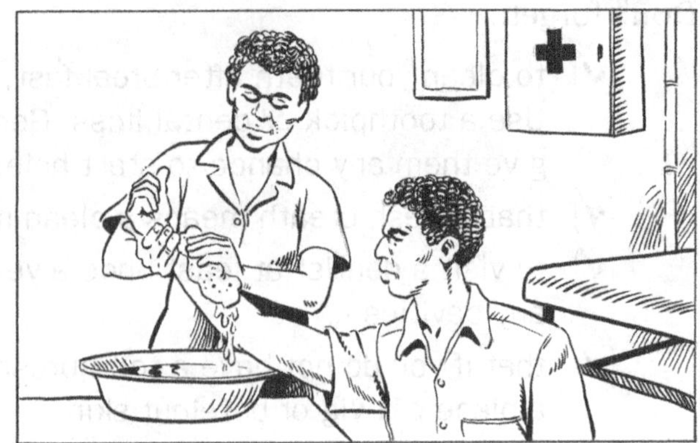

INFORMATION

Colds and influenza

Many people in towns and villages in Papua New Guinea need to know how to take care of themselves when faced with sicknesses affecting their health.

Two common illnesses that cannot be cured by medical treatments are colds and influenza (flu). They are both viral infections and the symptoms are very similar. Many people become confused with both illnesses, but severe symptoms are more likely with flu.

Symptoms/signs

- → Colds/flu: runny nose
- → Colds/flu: sneezing
- → Colds/flu: coughing
- → Colds/flu: headache
- → Colds: low-grade fever (slight fever)
- → Flu: fever
- → Colds: red, itchy eyes
- → Flu: fatigue, muscle aches
- → Colds: congested ears
- → Colds: sore throat

See your doctor or health worker if:

- → you have severe ear pain or trouble breathing or swallowing
- → you have a cough that is severe or lasts more than 10 days
- → you have mucus or sputum that is thick, smelly, or green or rust coloured
- → you have a fever with a temperature that stays above 38 degrees for three days
- → you have a history of severe heart or lung disease.

Home care tips for colds and flu

Encourage children to drink plenty of fluids, such as water and fruit juices and to avoid drinking coffee.

Take Panadol for fever and try chicken soup to soothe the throat.

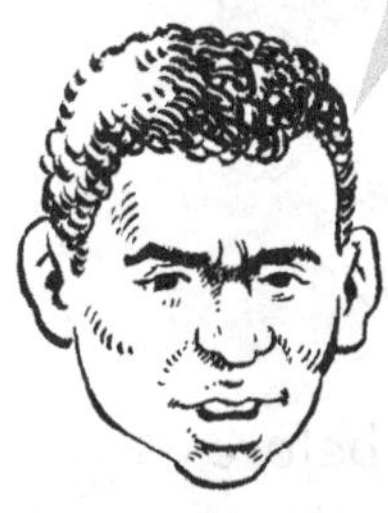

Reduce your activity and try to have a lot of bed rest. It is best to stay warm.

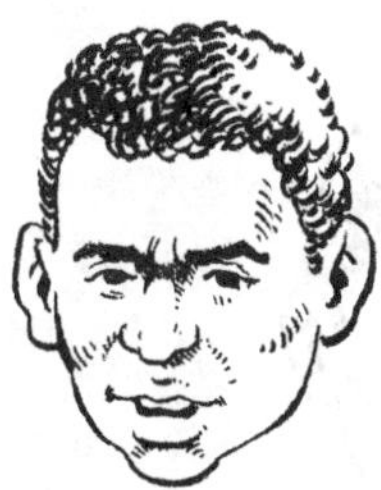

INFORMATION

Heartburn

Another common ailment that many young and old people experience is heartburn. Heartburn is a burning sensation and discomfort just below the breastbone.

Common contributors to heartburn are overeating, drinking alcohol and caffeine, taking aspirin, smoking tobacco and suffering from emotional stress.

Usually heartburn does not need a doctor unless the person is experiencing some intense discomfort. People having a heart attack sometimes think they have heartburn. If a person is experiencing shortness of breath, or pain in their jaw, right down the arm or in the back, seek medical attention immediately.

Symptoms/signs

Burning sensation and discomfort just below the breastbone, going up to the throat.

If heartburn lasts for more than three days and the person vomits black or bloody material, or has faeces that are black and tar-like, get medical attention urgently.

Home care tips for heartburn

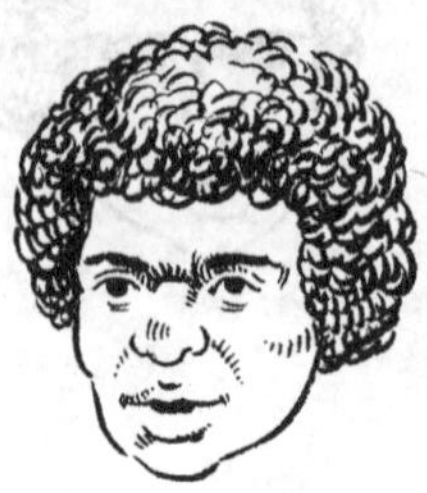

- Try to avoid vinegar, chocolate, oranges, lemons, grapefruits, pickles, peppermint and tomatoes.
- Avoid fatty foods, alcohol and caffeine, such as coffee and cola drinks.
- Stay mildly active for two hours after eating.

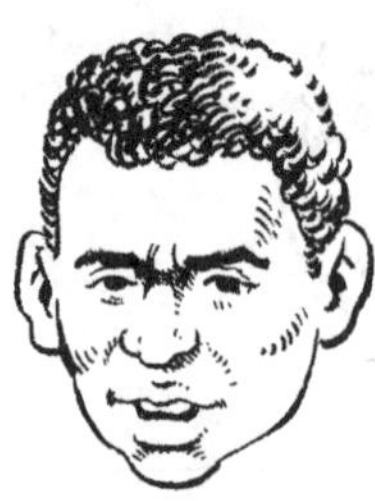

- An after-dinner walk may help the food to settle.
- Wait one or two hours after eating before lying down.
- Try to lie on your left side. If you need to rest, keep your shoulders elevated 30 to 60 centimetres above your hips (sitting up in bed with your head on two pillows).

Food additives

Many Papua New Guineans do not know what food additives are and the effect of these additives on health. Communities need to know about food additives.

Food additives are substances that food companies add to food to make them taste or look good.

Some additives are made from natural resources, such as soybeans and corn, to be used as food colouring. Others are man-made. Artificial additives can be produced more economically. Whether an additive is artificial or natural does not mean it is safe.

Is a natural additive safer because it is chemical free?

No. All foods, whether from the garden or the supermarket shelf, are made up of chemicals. For example, the vitamin C found in a pawpaw or an orange is identical to that made in a laboratory. Indeed, all things in the world consist of chemicals, such as carbon, hydrogen, nitrogen, oxygen and other elements. These elements are combined in various ways to produce starches, proteins, fats, water and vitamins found in foods.

 Cyanide

Cyanide is found naturally in a number of foods and plants, such as cassava roots. In villages throughout the country, cassava is grown for home consumption, feasts and other social gatherings.

How might I be exposed to cyanide?

- ☑ Breathing air, drinking water, touching soil, or eating foods containing cyanide. For example, if cassava is not cooked properly it contains cyanide.
- ☑ Smoking cigarettes and breathing smoke-filled air during fires are major sources of cyanide exposure.
- ☑ Breathing air near a hazardous waste site containing cyanide.
- ☑ Eating foods containing some cyanide, such as cassava roots, lima beans and almonds.
- ☑ Working in an industry where cyanide is produced, such as metal cleaning and photography.

How can cyanide affect my health?

Cyanide is very harmful especially when people are exposed to large amounts. Exposure to cyanide harms the brain and heart, and may cause coma and death.

Exposure to lower levels of cyanide for a long time may result in breathing difficulties, heart pains, vomiting, blood changes, headaches, and enlargement of the thyroid gland.

Skin contact with cyanide can produce irritation and sores.

If faced with a cyanide-related incident, go to the hospital for treatment and professional advice.

Alcohol

Drinking too much alcohol can make you fat. It is not food.

It takes about ten minutes for the alcohol to go from the mouth, to the stomach, to the intestine, to the bloodstream and to the heart. About 10 per cent of alcohol passes through the urine and breath, and 90 per cent is processed by the liver into carbon dioxide and hydrogen. It takes the liver an hour to process just one drink of alcohol.

People react in many different ways to alcohol. It depends on how much is drunk and also on how much your body can consume.

People who are drunk have problems with their judgement.

- Their sense of reason is affected unlike when they are sober.
- Their memory and self-control are affected. The more beer they drink, the more they lose control.

Regular drinking makes the body sick. It also contributes to loss of memory, abnormal heart disease and stomach ulcers and liver damage.

Say 'No' to friends when they try to persuade you to drink alcohol.

However if you drink, remember:

- respect people, and limit yourself
- drinking on an empty stomach is dangerous
- drink driving is dangerous
- drinking is not an excuse for bad behaviour
- get help from someone you trust when you are in trouble
- that young children learn from adults
- make sure to have a sober driver.

Remember alcohol may be the life of the party—but it might be the death of you.

Chapter 6 Why we need to exercise and stay fit

The role of exercise and fitness in our lives is very important. There are many benefits of being fit—it helps to develop both the body and the mind.

Exercising is a good way of minimising stress. It refreshes and relaxes the mind. There are two forms of exercising: physical and mental. Some physical exercises are: running, walking, jogging, swimming, skipping, and so on.

Mental exercise can be in the form of meditation, imagination, thinking and so on.

There are many psychological and social benefits to exercise and fitness too.

The benefits of exercise include the following:

Physical

- ☑ Increased energy, vitality and stamina
- ☑ Firm and toned muscles
- ☑ Weight control
- ☑ Improved circulation and skin tone
- ☑ Improved coordination and flexibility
- ☑ Improved posture and personal appearance
- ☑ Strengthening the heart

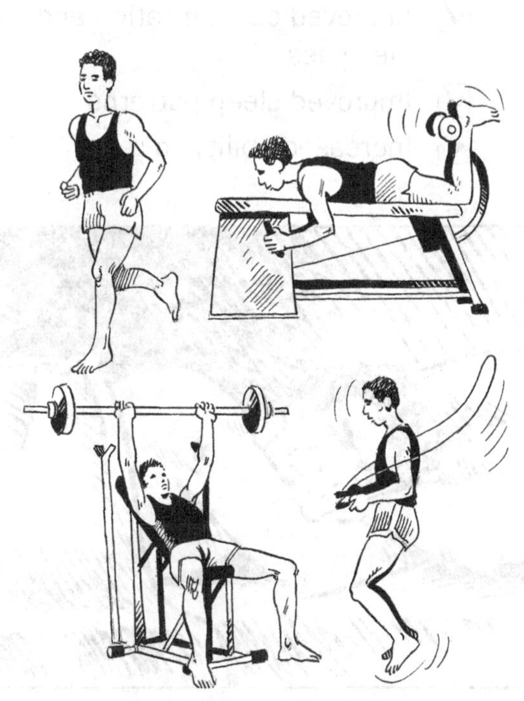

Social

- ☑ Meeting new people
- ☑ Developing friendships
- ☑ Learning to work as part of a team

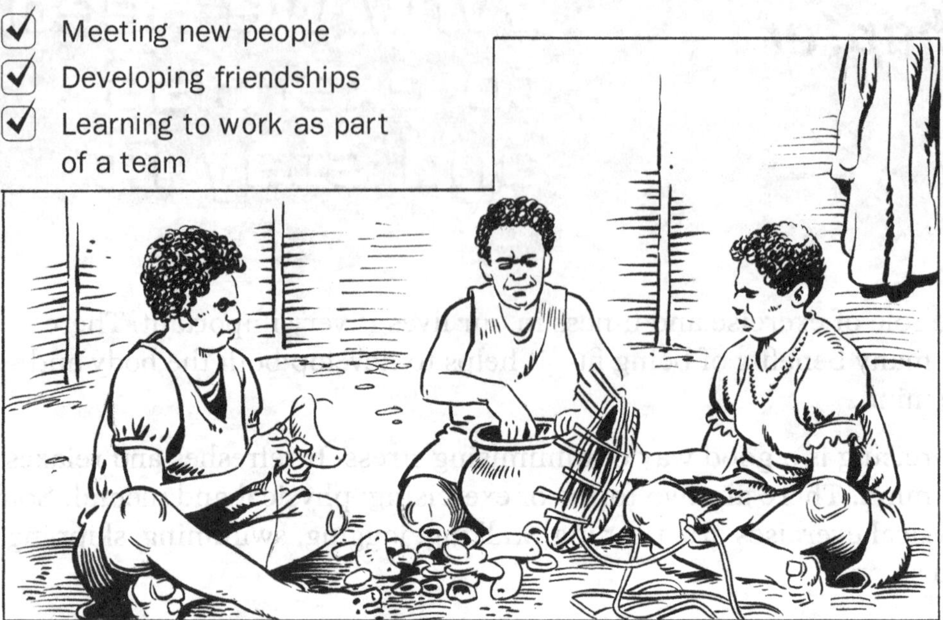

Mental

- ☑ Reduced stress levels
- ☑ Increased self-esteem and confidence
- ☑ Improved concentration and mental alertness
- ☑ Improved sleep patterns
- ☑ Increased ability to relax

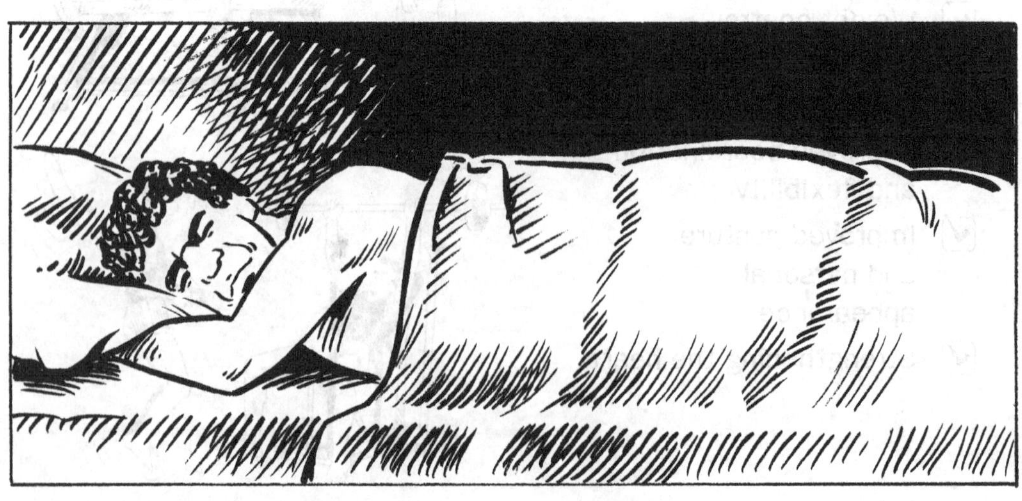

Most people have different views of exercise and how much is needed to maintain a good level of fitness.

What does it mean to be fit?

The term 'fitness' means more than having well-toned muscles and a slim body. It is having the energy to carry out everyday activities without becoming tired and still having enough energy in reserve to participate in leisure activities.

Fitness can be divided into two main groups:

- ☑ Health-related fitness, such as developing muscular strength, flexibility, body shape, and a healthy cardiovascular system. These are important because they help people to maintain a good level of health.
- ☑ Skill-related fitness, such as coordination, speed, power, balance, and agility. These skills are more specific to participating well in certain sports and can be improved with practice.

Activity 6·1

Write a schedule with a plan showing what exercise and how many should be done for each day. Do not forget to do warm up exercises before actually doing these exercises.

For example:

Activity	How many	Time
Push ups	15–20	3 Minutes
Sit ups	15–20	3 Minutes

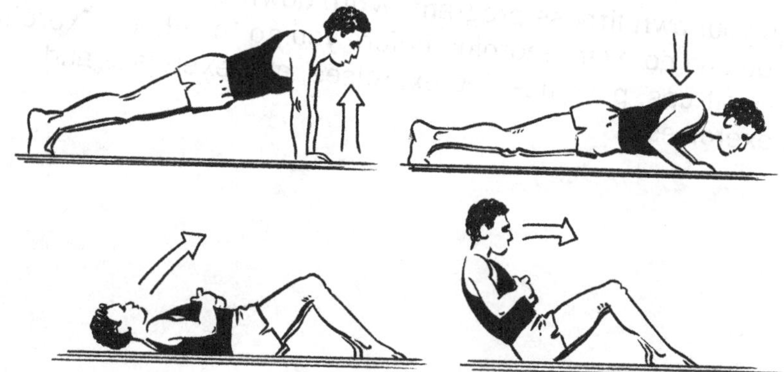

Play for exercise

Be active and exercise. Jump, climb, run, slide, swing, swim, garden or dance. This will keep you healthy.

Exercise your mind too by playing games like checkers, puzzles, hand strings. Learn honesty and self-discipline—you can do this by playing team games.

- ☑ Join other children in playing games.
- ☑ Play team games.
- ☑ Play in safe areas of your house and the surroundings.
- ☑ Take a rest after play or work. Sleep well!

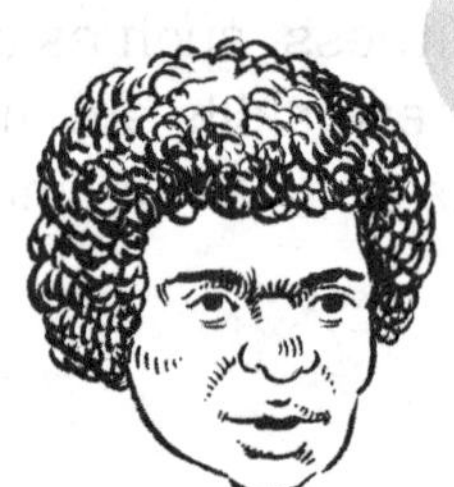

Activity 6·2

- Make a list of all the games that you enjoy playing. Next to each game indicate where this activity is normally played and at least two safety rules that should apply when playing this particular game.

Example :

Game	Venue	Safety Rule
Soccer	Soccer field	Wear shin guards
Rugby	Rugby field	Wear a mouth guard/ Wear head gear

- Design your own fitness program. Write down a list of exercises that you can do every morning before you go to school. Exercises such as sit ups, push ups, leg exercises, arm exercises and head exercises.

Avoid injury

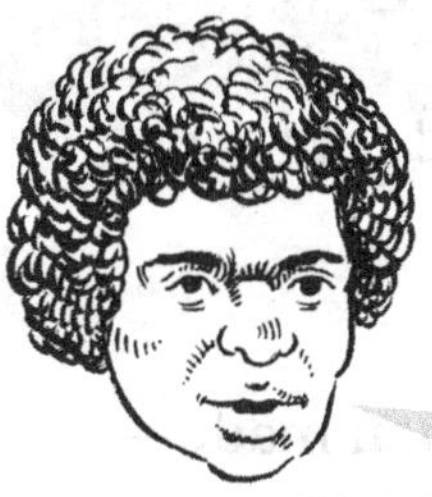

- Only swim in a river, lake, beach or swimming pool if you can swim well and have a friend with you. Ask your parents' permission.
- Be careful of dogs and other animals. Their bites can hurt you.
- Avoid toys that are pointed, sharp, or have a rough surface. These can give you a cut or wound.
- When you play inside the house, keep away from cooking pots, the clothes iron, stairs and windows.
- Be careful with a broken electric wire. Inform your elders as soon as you see a naked wire.

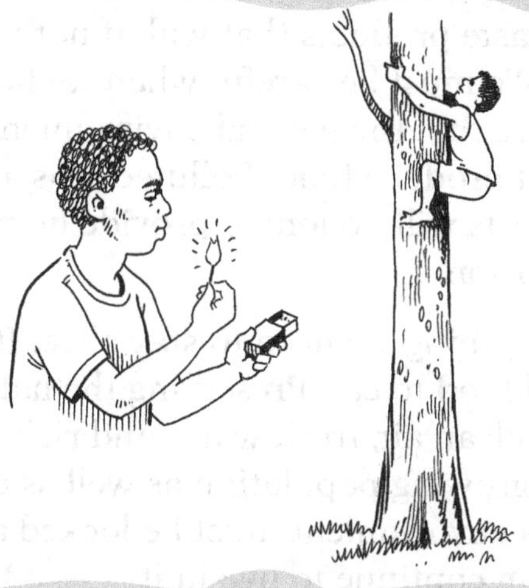

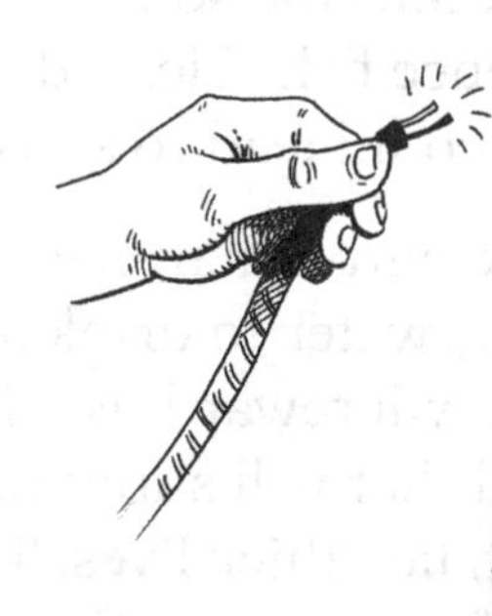

- To avoid hurting yourself, be careful and avoid playing in places that are dangerous.
- When you play outside the house, choose somewhere away from the street, like a courtyard, or gardens. If you can, play in a public park, your school grounds, or a sports field.
- Before you cross the street, always look right and left to check that there are no vehicles coming.
- Be careful when climbing trees.
- Remember: play where it is safe.

Chapter 7 How to plan for a healthy environment

Conservation means using your environment (natural and man made—that is everything that surrounds you and the world in which you live) wisely and planning for the future. Human survival depends on resources such as enough food, clean air and water, sufficient shelter, clothing and fuel. However, as the population increases more and more of these resources are needed. More people will need fish from the sea, more timber from the forests and crops and minerals from the land. This will in turn produce more waste products that will, if not managed wisely, pollute the environment. We must be careful when we build man-made environments that we ensure that the natural environment is not damaged. An infertile soil will not produce food. Polluted seas and rivers will not produce fish. Cleared forests will no longer provide homes for animals and could lead to soil erosion.

Our natural environment has everything we need to stay alive. It has air to breathe, water to drink and food to eat. Preserving the natural environment will reward us with clean air, fresh water and rich land for growing food that will support a growing population as well as enable us to live longer, healthier lives. This environment must be looked after so that we and future generations can continue to live in it.

The consequences of polluting the natural environment include air, water and land pollution. Polluting the environment causes health problems.

Air pollution

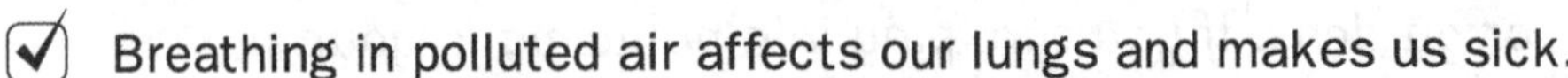

- ☑ Breathing in polluted air affects our lungs and makes us sick.
- ☑ Burning bushes/trees/rubbish releases toxic chemicals into the air that also affect our lungs and are irritating to the eyes.

Water pollution

- ☑ Chemicals released from mining activities into the river pollute and contaminate the same water that people use for washing and drinking. This is the same river where people catch fish to eat.
- ☑ Rivers and canals become breeding grounds for disease-producing germs when industrial and household wastes are dumped in them. These germs can give you diarrhoea, typhoid fever, stomach and liver sickness and food poisoning.

Land pollution

The use of too many fertilisers, pesticides and other chemicals destroy the soil, plant and animal life, and may lead to fatal diseases. Pesticides are poisons which can enter water or food webs. When an animal feeds or drinks, the chemicals enter the body. People then eat these animals and can be exposed to these poisons.

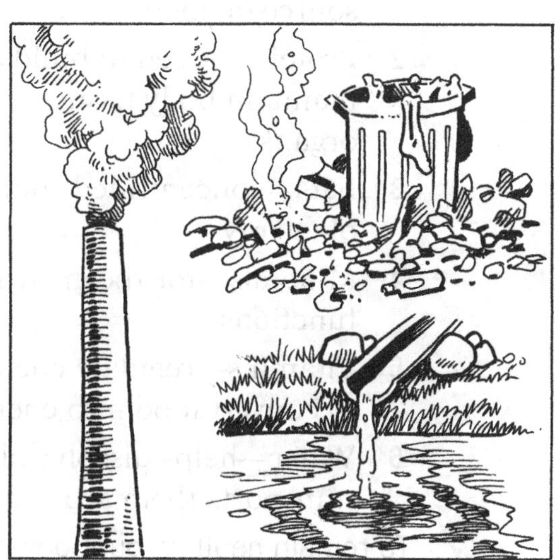

Everyone helps to make a healthy environment

At home, everyone should:

- dispose of rubbish properly in covered containers,
- avoid dumping rubbish in river, canals or ponds, and
- bury garbage that cannot be reused or disposed of in another way

In your community, everyone should:

- Organise activities to protect the environment. Keep it a healthy place to live in.
- Plant trees and vegetables on vacant land and avoid using chemical fertilisers or pesticides.

What have we learnt?

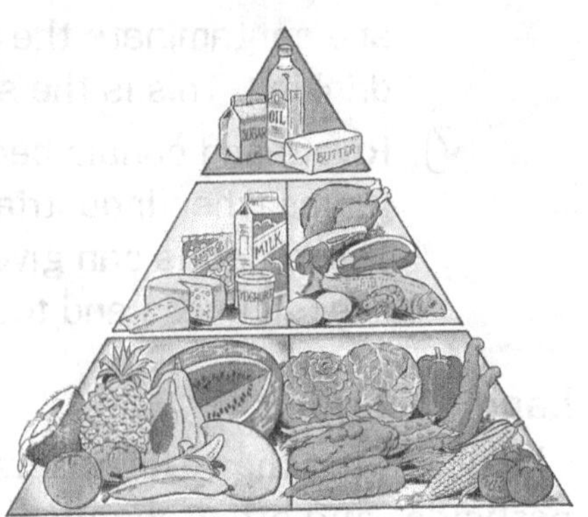

- ☑ The body needs food and energy. Food contains nutrients that help the body to function properly.
- ☑ There are six major nutrients.
  1. Carbohydrates—the major source of energy
  2. Proteins—used to build and maintain body tissues and organs
  3. Fats—concentrated source of energy
  4. Minerals—for the growth and maintenance of body functions

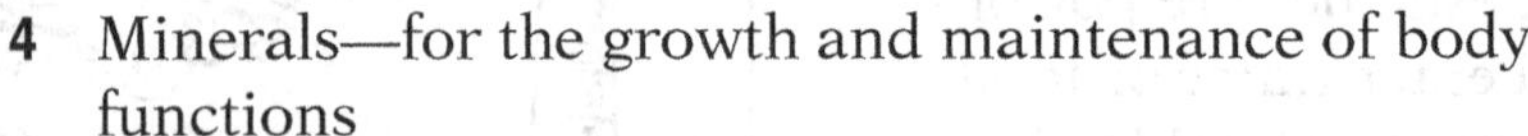

  5. Vitamins—regulate chemical reactions that allow our body to convert food into energy and tissues
  6. Water—helps dissolve all the nutrients our body needs and transports them around the body
- ☑ To remain healthy, our body needs a balanced diet of the six nutrients.
- ☑ An improper or inadequate diet can lead to a number of diseases.
- ☑ To keep our body healthy we need to maintain personal hygiene.
- ☑ A clean water supply is essential for people's health and hygiene.
- ☑ A healthy lifestyle means that everyone must live in a clean environment, have a healthy diet and have good personal hygiene.
- ☑ Exercise and fitness are very important to develop both body and mind.

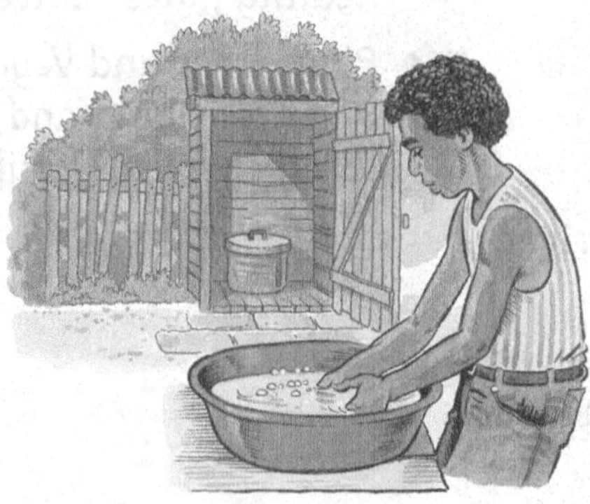

Glossary

additives
something added as an ingredient to keep food fresh or improve its texture, colour or provide a beneficial effect

alcohol
an intoxicating colourless liquid found in wine, beer, gin

amoebic dysentery
intestinal disease varies from acute to severe dysentery with fever, chills and bloody diarrhoea

anaemia
lack of red blood cells in the body to carry oxygen to the tissues for the body to function normally

antibiotics
substance produced by a bacteria or fungus that destroys or weakens germs

artificial
not natural; made by human skill or labour

bacteria
very tiny and simple organism that can be seen through a microscope

calcium
a soft silvery-white element that is the main component of bones

carbohydrate
a substance made by green plants in sunlight from carbon dioxide and water. Carbohydrates are made from carbon, hydrogen and oxygen. Sugar and starch are carbohydrates. Carbohydrates comprise a major class of foods for animals

chemical
any substance made or used in chemistry

contaminate
to make impure or dirty, which may cause infection or other problems

cyanide
a metallic salt used in the manufacture of plastics and insecticides and in the extraction of gold ore. Also found in uncooked cassava

defecate
passing of faeces

dehydration
the result of lack of water in the body or removal of water from other substances

diarrhoea
a condition of excessively frequent and loose bowel movements

diet
the usual kind of food and drink for a person or animal

fat
oily substance found in animal bodies

fertiliser
any substance, organic or inorganic, that makes soil richer when it is spread over or put into soil

fever
when a person's body is too hot, sometimes with sweating and sometimes with dry skin. The pulse is usually faster than normal. Fever comes with many illnesses

flu
influenza, an infectious viral disease

food-borne diseases
diseases that can be spread through contaminated food

food poisoning
result from eating food containing certain bacteria, bacterial toxins or chemicals

germ
any micro-organism (for instance bacterium, virus, protozoan), especially one that causes disease

high-energy food
food high in energy, such as fat and sugar, needed by the body to function normally

kwashiorkor
a fatal condition related to a diet lacking in protein

liver
large reddish-brown organ that produces bile; aids in food absorption; breaks down waste matter in blood and produces blood proteins

malaria
a disease characterised by fever and sweats caused by a bite from a mosquito. The mosquito can pass malaria from one person to another

malnutrition
a condition when someone is poorly nourished. People suffer from malnutrition because of eating the wrong kinds of food as well as lack of food

marasmic
wasting away of the body resulting from malnutrition

meningitis
a serious infectious disease in which the membranes surrounding the brain or spinal cord are inflamed

minerals
substances, neither plant nor animal, that the body requires for good health

morbidity
the proportion of sickness in a certain group or locality

mortality
loss of life; frequency of death

mucus
a slimy substance secreted by the mucous membranes of the body

natural
something produced by nature; not man made

nutrition
the processes by which living things take in food and use it

pesticides
substances or chemicals used to kill insects

pneumonia
when the lungs are inflamed resulting in coughs, high fever and pain

pollute
to make physically impure or dirty; contaminate

protein-energy malnutrition
occurs when the diet is low in both proteins and calories

proteins
one of the substances containing nitrogen, hydrogen, carbon and oxygen, that is a necessary part of animals and plants

staple food
food that contains high amounts of carbohydrates and forms the basis of meals

toxic
poison

tuberculosis
a disease affecting the lungs. It is contagious and spreads by breathing in droplets in the air

underweight
having too little weight; not to the required weight

vegetables
the part of a plant used for food

vitamin A deficiency
lack of vitamin A in the body that can lead to night blindness

vitamin C
vitamin found in citrus fruits and pawpaw; prevents and cures scurvy

vitamins
any one of certain special substances necessary for the normal growth and proper nourishment of the body

water
a liquid that is necessary for all living things and is also a nutrient

water-borne diseases
diseases that can be spread through contaminated water